ROGERS' SCHOOL OF HERBAL MEDICINE

VOLUME NINE:

THE BRAIN

ROBERT DALE ROGERS RH (AHG)

COVER
Top: Sunflower
Middle: Periwinkle
Bottom Left: Henbane flowers
Bottom Right: Magic Mushrooms

This book is for educational purposes only. The suggestions, recipes and historical information are not meant to replace a medical advisor. The author assumes no liability for unwise or unsafe usage by readers of this book.

For those interested in using herbal medicine, seek the advice of a professional.

TABLE OF CONTENTS

ALBIZIA	1
ASHWAGANDHA	3
BACOPA	8
BUFFALO BERRY	11
BURNET	183
CALAMUS	23
CANBY'S LOVAGE	41
CLUBMOSS	44
COMB TOOTH	118
COW ITCH	132
DAFFODIL	62
FABA BEAN	75
FIG MARIGOLD	127
GINKGO BILOBA	91
GOTU KOLA	98
HENBANE	104
ICE PLANT	127
JERUSALEM ARTICHOKE	204
LION'S MANE	118
MUCUNA	132
NARCISSUS	62
PANAEOLUS	152
PERIWINKLE	139
PSILOCYBE	157
SAGE	167
SALAD BURNET	183
SNOWDROP	194
STROPHARIA	157
SUNFLOWER	203
VELVET BEAN	132

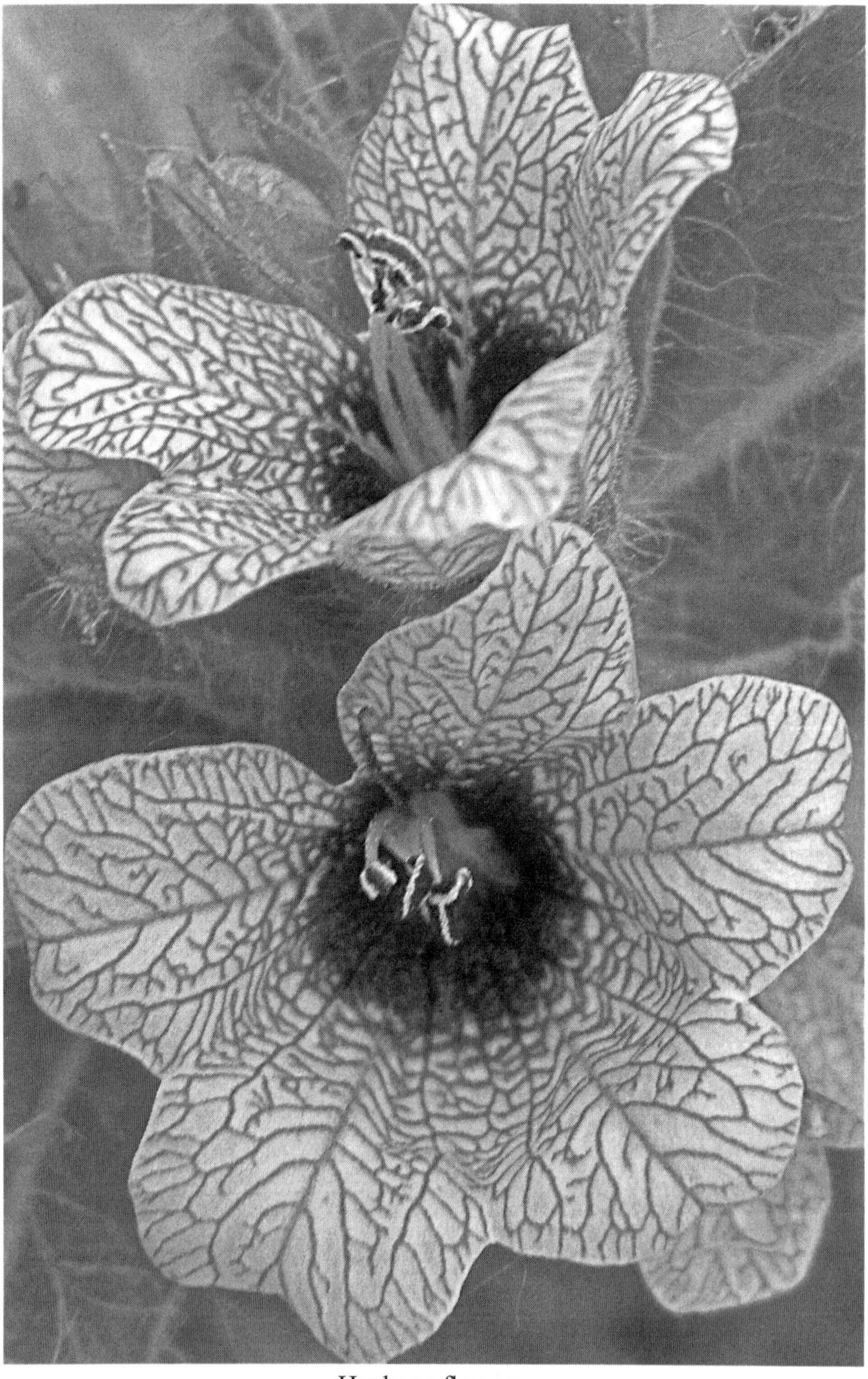

Henbane flowers

THE BRAIN

The Brain is a wonderful and complex part of the body. In fact, we often talk about mind-body connection, as if the thinking and feeling part of use is distinct from our physicality.

This is, of course, untrue, and a concept that has led us down the biomedical model that treats disease and symptoms.

I could not even begin to present the various named lobes of the brains, and their various associated connections in this small contribution.

Rather, I am going to follow a novel concept by Dr. Eric R. Braverman, outlined in his book, *The Edge Effect*. The book is highly recommended to all students of herbal medicine.

Braverman suggests that the four domains of brain health are memory, attention, personality and temperament, and physical health.

"The difference between a resourceful mind and senility is only one hundred milliseconds of brain speed, which means you have fewer than a hundred milliseconds to lose over the course of your life... By the time our thinking is slowed to four hundred milliseconds, we can no longer process logical thoughts...These medical, neurological and psychiatric conditions related to loss of brain speed can cascade into obesity, anxiety, depression, psychosis, multiple sclerosis and Parkinson's disease; 50% of Americans will have developed some degree of impairment from dementia or Alzheimer's disease by age eight, and 80 percent will do so by ninety."

It is important to add the enteric nervous system (ENS) to the discussion at this point. Under the Nervous System, we looked at the central and autonomic nervous systems. The ENS operates independently of the brain and spinal cord, but it does receive and act on information received from the central nervous system via the vagus nerve (parasympathetic) and prevertebral ganglia (sympathetic). It is often called the "second brain" due to some one hundred million neurons, similar in number to those in the spinal cord.

It is embedded in the gastro-intestinal lining and makes use of more than 30 neurotransmitters, including acetylcholine, dopamine and serotonin. In fact, more than 90% of the body's serotonin and 50% of the body's dopamine is found in the gut.

Hence, the importance of digestive health to mental health. There is also a heart brain. See Cardiovascular book for more information.

We are born with roughly one hundred billion neurons, and in turn, each neuron has thousands of dendrites that connect up our electrical system. Neurons come close to each other, but are separated by a synaptic gap. The axon of a neuron relies on neuro-chemicals to cross this gap and connect with the dendrite of another neuron.

The brain generates the largest electrical charge in the body, and delivers it via voltage, speed, rhythm and synchrony. The latter come in the form of alpha, beta, theta and delta waves, each one balancing the other throughout the day.

The four primary neuro-chemicals involved are dopamine, acetylcholine, GABA and serotonin. I know there are others, just bear with me.

Beta brain waves, associated with alertness, occur when in the frontal lobe, when dopamine is present. Dopamine works like a natural amphetamine and controls energy, excitement, motivation, as well as bodily functions such as blood pressure, metabolism and digestion.

It helps generate the electricity that controls voluntary movement, intelligence, abstract thought, long-term planning and personality traits.

The beta state begins to predominate at about the age of thirteen, and is associated with reason and analysis. This helps us to express ourselves and give our intuition direction and form.

It should be noted that those individuals dominated by beta have a mental pattern of constant, low-power chatter. It is a state of questioning rather than action, and not being tuned into intuition. Low amplitude beta states lead to living according to belief systems.

Its by-product is adrenaline. Lack of dopamine can lead to addictive behaviour, obesity, exhaustion and, of course, Parkinson's disease.

When deficient, the body naturally increases levels of cortisol, produced by the adrenal glands.

When dopamine is present in excessive amounts, violent controlled behavior including reckless driving, sexual assault and other criminal activity may be present. Cocaine attaches itself to dopamine transporters, preventing re-absorption. Crack cocaine targets the ventral tegmental area of the brain.They tend to crave carbohydrates. Dopamine types represent about 17% of the population. Sources of dopamine precursors are ginseng, nettles, red clover, milk thistle, fenugreek, dandelion, peppermint and beets.

Alpha brain waves help the brain understand and react to sensory input. They are produced in the parietal lobes, and associated with acetylcholine, controlling brain speed. In a sense, acetylcholine is a lubricant, helping act as a building block for the myelin sheath that surrounds the neurons, like plastic or rubber covers an electrical wire. This insulation makes sure the signal does not lose strength until it reaches its destination.

By the age of seven, the alpha wave state begins to predominate, and children become indoctrinated into expectations of family and society. Alpha waves operate at seven to thirteen cycles per second. Alpha is a state through which the subconscious mind interprets information and experiences which occurred before birth and during infancy. These may include phobias, complexes and positive affirmations. This state influences how information from other sources, including transpersonal self, are interpreted and expressed. As the child moves to thirteen, theta becomes less dominant and the body changes form that is less capable of expressing functions of higher self.

Acetylcholine out of balance can lead to language disorders, childhood learning disabilities, and of course Alzheimer's disease. In deficient states, they tend to crave rich, and fatty foods, and may binge on sweets or caffeine.

Phosphatidyl serine is a helpful supplement for deficient states.

In excess, this type gives too much of themselves to point of being masochistic. They may feel as if the world is taking advantage of them, or paranoia and isolation take place.

Acetylcholine types makes up about 17% of the population.

Many herbs inhibit acetylcholinesterase that breaks down this compound. Angelica seed, clubmoss, wild bergamot and rosemary are few examples.

Theta brain waves are associated with drowsiness and are related to GABA (gamma-aminobutyric acid), produced in the temporal lobes. These lobes help balance the frontal lobes which govern personality, and the parietal lobes controlling thinking and acting. GABA is the brain's natural tranquilizer, giving calmness to mind, body and spirit. There are about ten known GABA type receptors in the brain.

Theta waves are involved in the production of endorphins, the feel good hormone associated with "runner's high". They can be produced during exercise and sexual intercourse. An imbalance can lead to headaches, hypertension, heart palpitations, low sex drive and seizures. Almost 50% of the world's population is a GABA type. This is a good thing, as GABA in balance is stable, consistent, social and concerned with well-being of others. You are a team player, and rarely have broad swings of emotions or outbursts of anger. GABA deficiency can cause frequent bowel movements, due to its effect on the rhythm of the intestinal tract.

When suffering chronic pain, the deficient GABA type may turn to marijuana, alcohol or narcotics. In hippocampus, it helps with orientation of time and space.

When present in excess, it can lead to people expending energy seeking love and opportunities to take care of others, at neglect of their own health. Too little GABA can leave one feeling tired throughout the day. The theta state generally occurs at four to seven cycles per second and predominates from birth until about seven years of age. This is the time children have the greatest capacity to express themselves uniquely, because they do not have enough reasoning power to question themselves. Theta is a non-judgemental state, with little editing of what is observed and experienced. The brain, of course, records everything happening in their environment.

The body makes use of L-glutamine to produce GABA. One of our richest vegetable sources is red cabbage, particularly when fermented as in sauerkraut. L-theanine, from green tea, is an excellent inducer of GABA. Take 100-250 mg two or three times daily.

Delta waves are related to the production of serotonin and the occipital lobes that control the visual process. Serotonin provides a soothing, nourishing feeling and when levels are adequate, sleep is deep and peaceful, food is enjoyable and though patterns are appropriate. When out of balance, depression, hormonal imbalance, including PMS, as well as eating and sleeping disorders can be present. About 17% of the population are serotonin types. They exhibit great eye-hand coordination when in balance, but can become risk takers when deficient. A distain for order and structure and a love of independence can create undue hardships. Delta waves occur at one to four cycles per second. Infants one to two years old are in predominantly delta-theta state, when the mind and body are in harmony.

Too much serotonin can make you extremely nervous, making you vulnerable to criticism, afraid of being disliked, and becoming hesitant or distracted. In the extreme, one can be extremely shy and withdrawn, suffering issues of self worth, sadness and desperate need for interpersonal relationship. Anorexia and bulimia are related to serotonin deficiency. Too little serotonin can produce insomnia and night sweats. Sources of serotonin precursors are oats, angelica, burdock, dandelion, ginger, wild yam, black cohosh and marijuana.

It is important to remember that serotonin receptors, particularly 5-$HT2_a$ is not just found in the nervous system, but also in our platelets, the cardiovascular system, our enteric nervous system, in mast cells, fibroblasts, on neurons of peripheral nervous system and in human monocytes.

Stephen Buhner, in *Plant Intelligence*, reminds us. "Serotonin, and these kinds of receptors, are not limited to human beings however. They are ubiquitous throughout the living systems of the planet: in animals, insects and plants."

To further complicate (or clarify) the issue, let us look at the corpus callosum. It helps connect the left and right hemispheres of the brain. As we know, left-brained individuals are more analytical, thinking and rely on practical skills. They are well-organized and see things as part of patterns or sequences. Left brainers are GABA dominant, and make sure that everything is in good working order, right-side up and all that.

Right-brained individuals focus on feelings, intuition and are more socially active, spontaneous, and empathic. They are dominated by acetylcholine, controlling creativity and speed. They are very sensitive to feelings of others and are a joy to be around.

Aspberger's and various ADD classifications may benefit from herbal supplementation. In the case of the former, there may be strong head brain connection and compromised gut-brains. That is, both Aspberger's and ADD individuals have a high incidence of intestinal dysbiosis, and elevated levels of gluten and casein sensitivity. Due to "leaky gut syndrome", there may be issues of the heart, with emotional need for protection due to intensity of feelings.

The leaky brain syndrome can lack speech or hearing filters, resulting in anxiety.

There are three main classes of anti-depressant medications.

The first, Monamine oxidase inhibitors, enhance norepinephrine, serotonin and dopamine and are an older class of drugs that are the most dangerous and least prescribed today. They inhibit the reuptake of tyramine, which can result in acute hypertension and can interact with wine, cheese and other tyramine rich foods.

The second are tricyclic anti-depressants, that stimulate norepinephrine and serotonin in the brain. Known as monoamines, they must be inactivated and re-uptaken by secreting cells. Known as TRIs, they block the reuptake, allowing them to remain in body for longer.

The newest class is the SSRIs, or selective serotonin reuptake inhibitors. This includes Prozac, Luvox, Paxil, Celexa, and Zoloft. They work by blocking serotonin re-absorption. They prolong the effects of serotonin, with enhanced sense of well being.

All three have a long list of side effects, and expectant mothers need to avoid use during the third trimester, due to adverse effects on child after birth.

Now, let us look at some herbs and mushrooms useful for brain health.

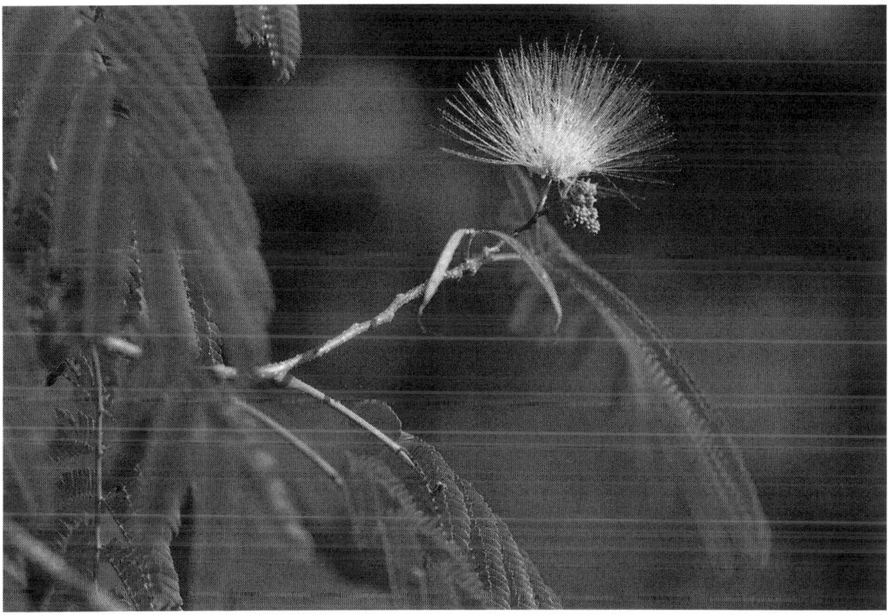

Bastard tamarind (*Albizia julibrissin*)

ALBIZIA
(*A. julibrissin* Durazzini**)**
PARTS USED- flower, bark

Albizia, the Tree of Happiness, is found in temperate part of the United States as well as its native regions of China, Korea and Japan.

In Mandarin, the flowers are known as **HUAN HUA**, and the bark **HE HUAN PI**. In Cantonese, the flower is **HAP FUN FA**, the bark **HAP FUN PEI**. They are known as the Happiness Herb and Collective Happiness Bark, respectively.

It was first recorded in the 2nd century in the Shen Nong Ben Cao as a calmative and mood tonic, for those suffering loss of a loved one, or similar calamity.

According to Michael Tierra, "the bark is thought to 'anchor' the spirit, while the flowers 'lighten' it."

Albizia seeds were placed on a herbarium sheet in the Natural History Museum in 1793. It was fire bombed in 1940 and when water was sprayed on the ashes they woke up and germinated.

MEDICINAL

CONSTITUENTS- albiticon, beta sitosterol, amyrin, 3,4,7, trihydroxyflavone, spinasteryl glucoside, machaerinic, lactone, acaci acid, and various saponins, tannins, methyl esters.

Albizia is thought to enhance all aspects of neurotransmitter secretion and regulation.

There are few studies on the herb. One study of the flower extract found increased pentobarbital-induced sleeping time in mice. Kang et al, *J Ethnopharm* 2000 71 321-23.

The bark is a powerful anti-oxidant, based on methanol extracts. Jung et al, *Arch Pharm Res* 2003 26:6 458-62.

In TCM, albizia bark is considered sweet, dry and astringent, with neutral energy, entering the heart and liver meridians. It is used primarily for insomnia, memory, irritability and angry feelings due to constrained emotions. The bark is used for external trauma and injury, promoting blood circulation, reducing pain and swelling and regeneration of broken bones.

It is specific for heart yin deficiency with liver yang rising, a picture of anxiety, irritability, restlessness, tightness in chest and insomnia.

Symptoms may include paranoia, phobias, neurocardiac disorders and apprehension.

It is a detoxifying resolvent in cases of boils, abscesses and carbuncles, including lung abscess with vomiting of pus.

Michael Tierra writes. "As well as giving albizia to many patients suffering from acute and chronic depression and anxiety, I've also given it to those who complain of high stress, with noticed marked improvement even after a single day of use…Albizia is a good choice for probably greater than 50% of those who are presently taking a pharmaceutical drug. At a mere fraction of the price, albizia is devoid of the adverse side effects of the drugs and can be easily stopped at anytime."

The flowers are used for same heart syndrome as bark, and like it help relieve abdominal pain and spasmodic lumps due to Liver stagnation due to emotional blockage. The flower tea helps improve memory and promote sleep. Both bark and flower are excellent shen stabilizers, but the flower is much strong mood elevating (shen-lifting) herb.

The herb is oxytocic, and therefore contraindicated in pregnancy.

The bark combines well with reishi, white peony root, calamus root, goji berry, schisandra berry and licorice root as a shen tonic. This will calm, soothe and uplift the spirit, and help those who have suffered heartbreak, or worry excessively, or are mentally or emotionally exhausted.

RECIPES

TINCTURE- one half teaspoon three times daily, up to a teaspoon or a tablespoon in severe cases. The tincture is made from either dry flower or bark at 1:5 and 40% alcohol.

DECOCTION- 10-16 grams of a 1:2 bark decoction. Drink cool.

INFUSION- One tablespoon of dried flowers to one pint of boiled water. Steep for ten minutes, cool. Drink 4-6 ounces several times daily.

CAUTION- Do not use concurrently with any of MAOs, SSRIs or tricyclic anti-depressants. Do not use without presence of heart Qi constraint.

ASHWAGANDHA
WINTER CHERRY
INDIAN GINSENG
(*Withania somnifera* [L.] Dunal.**)**
(*Physalis somnifera* L.**)**
PART USED- root, berries, leaves

Ashwagandha is a small, evergreen member of the Solanaceae family. In Sanskrit the name means "odor of the horse", due to sweaty horse odor of fresh root. This is suggestive of the sexual potency of a stallion, and thus its use in treating infertility, and impotence.

Somnifera is from the Latin meaning "sleep-inducer", due to its use in relieving stress and help in insomnia.

The root has been used as a diuretic and in various aphrodisiac formulas over time. It is worth noting that the fresh root was traditionally boiled in milk to leach out undesirable constituents.

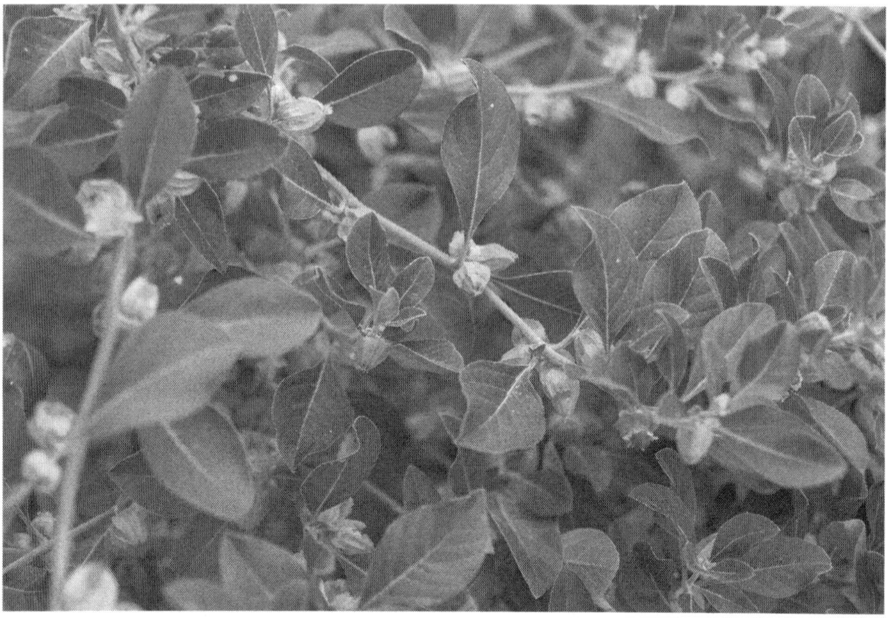

Indian Ginseng

The berries were used to coagulate milk, and produce cheese.

Native to Asia, into India, as well as Africa and southern Europe, the shrub has moved into the southern United States.

In West African folk medicine, the root and leaves have been used for fevers, and rheumatic pain. The Sotho use it as a ritual plant against witchcraft, and anthelmintic. A decoction of the root is used to tone the uterus of women who regularly miscarry, and to remove retained contraceptive products.

In Somalia, the root decoction is given to children for fever, nightmares and disturbed sleep.

The Xhosa and Pedi use the fresh plant to disinfect meat suspected infected with anthrax. In southern Africa, it is used for "black-gall sickness", asthma, bronchitis, and various venereal diseases.

MEDICINAL

CONSTITUENTS- ergostane-type steroidal lactones including withaferin A, withanolides, with a-dienolides, withasomniferols and withanone withanolides; tropane alkaloids including withanine, tropine and pseudo-tropine; piperidine alkaloids anaferine, anahygrine, and isopelletierine; and cucohygrine, a pyrrolidine alkaloid.

The herb is considered an adaptogenic tonic, and may have been best placed in the book on Adaptogens. It has been used for over three millennia to help restore energy, strength, memory and counteract stress on the mind and body. It helps to calm the mind and promote inner peace and tranquility.

A good review of its uses looked at 58 articles and concluded the herb is beneficial as an anti-inflammatory, anti-tumor, anti-stress, antioxidant, immune modulator; and helping benefit the central nervous system. Mishra LC et al, *Altern Med Rev* 2000 5:4 334-346.

Other studies suggest anti-anxiety and anti-depressant activity comparable to lorazepam and imipramine. The root is excellent when there is depression present, with anxiety or panic attacks, a racing mind, exhaustion and insomnia.

In one double-blind, randomized, placebo-controlled trial of 64 subjects with a history of chronic stress, one capsule containing 300 mg of ashwangandha extract was given to one group and placebo capsule to other.

Treatment was for sixty days, and the serum cortisol levels were substantially reduced in herbal group. Chandrasekhar K et al, *Indian J Psycho Med* 2012 34:3 255-62.

An open label trial of 100 breast cancer patients, given the herb at dose of 2 grams every eight hours through chemotherapy, helped reduce fatigue. Biswal et al, *Integ Can Ther* 2013 12:4.

It is excellent for memory and learning and will help to gradually improve libido after a month or so. In a study of 75 normal healthy fertile men and 75 undergoing fertility screening, the latter showed improvements in levels of T, LH, FSH and PRL. All are good indicators of semen quality. Ahmad MK et al, *Fertil Steril* 2010 94:3 989-96.

Progressive degenerative cerebellar ataxia is a difficult to treat disease that severely affects balance. A small study on ten patients found ayurvedic therapies, including massage, steam baths and ashawagandha (500 mg) capsules three time daily for one month, showed statistically significant improvement in balance of patients. Sriranjini SJ et al, *Neurol India* 2009 57:2 166-71.

One interesting study found the herb reversed Alzheimer's disease (AD) pathology in transgenic mice. It mediated through up-regulation of liver lipoprotein receptor-related protein. This is a unique mechanism for clearance of beta-amyloid peptides, helping reverse behavioral deficits and pathology seen in AD. Shegal N et al, *Proc Natl Acad Sci USA* 2012 109:9 3510-5.

Inhibition of acetylcholinesterase is one approach in treatment or prevention of AD. In one study, withanolide A was found to be a valuable ligand molecule in treatment and prevention of AD pathologies. Grover et al, *J Biomol Struct Dyn* 2012 29:4 651-62.

Withanamides A & C showed protection of PC-12 cells, rat neuronal cells, from beta amyloid induced cell damage. It is suggested the withanamides prevent fibril formation, but more information and *in vivo* efficacy remain to be tested. Jayaprakasam B et al, *Phytother Res* 2010 24:6 859-63.

A randomized, double-blind, placebo-controlled pilot trial study on patients of schizophrenia shows promise for this difficult condition. Agnihotri AP et al, *Ind J Pharmacol* 2013 45:4 417-8.

Verbal working memory in bipolar disorders has improved in randomized, placebo-controlled trial of 60 patients. Chengappa KNR et al, *J Clin Psychiatry* 2013 74(11).

When ashwagandha was added to beta amyloid and HIV-1 infected samples, their toxic effects were neutralized. Kurapati KR et al, *PLoS One* 2013 8:10.

HOMEOPATHY

Sadness, low spirits, indifferent, cannot collect thoughts. Lascivious dreams with emissions. Confused with dull headache, buzzing in head, vertigo when standing or walking. The eyes are painful in morning, with weak sight and blue margins.

Whizzing in ears, face pale, and flushes of heat. Pressure in stomach, with drowsiness, nausea and vomiting.

Frequent desire and burning urine. Spermatorrhoea with emissions at night and during stool. Palpitations, pain in back, and great debility in extremities.

DOSE- low potency. Symptoms from Dr. B. Canbooly in Hom Rec 1922 volume 37.

BOTANICA POETICA
Ashwaganda
Withania somnifera
Here we have from India
And herb that will rejuvenate
It's been used for centuries
And your nerves, it can sedate
Stimulate your appetite
Anti-inflammatory if you need
Ashwaganda helps with stress
And it helps you fall asleep
Toxic leaves and toxic berries
A nightshade to use with care
Dry the root before you use it
In small amounts you'll better fare
It's an herb for nervous tension
An antioxidant as well
Put a poultie on your pimples
You'll be looking oh so swell
Give Ashwaganda to your boyfriend
If he needs a little boost
An aphrodisiac and tonic
You might find that in this root!
SYLVIA CHATROUX MD

RECIPES

CAPSULES- 300-500 mg capsules two to four times daily.

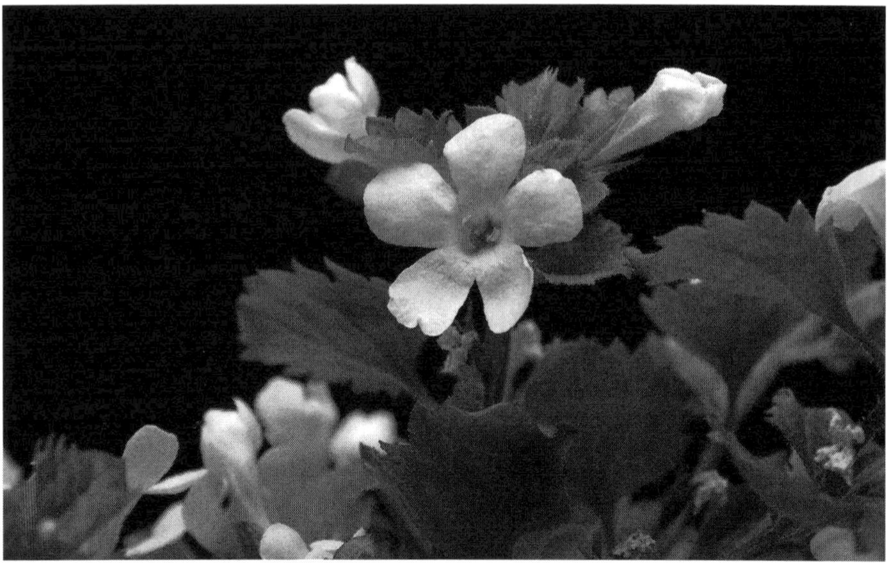

Bacopa flowers

WATER HYSSOP
(*Bacopa rotundifolia* [Michx] Wettst.)
BACOPA
INDIAN PENNYWORT
(*B. monniera* [L.] Pennell)

Bacopa is the Latin form of an aboriginal name used for a related plant by natives of French Guinea. Rotundifolia means round-leaved.

Water Hyssop is a succulent, aquatic perennial found in mud-bottomed pools of water in southern Alberta.

The most famous medicinal member of the genus is Brahmi (*B. monniera*), a memory enhancer from the Ayurvedic tradition of India. The plant is known as Thyme-leaved Gratiola, Bamb, Lonika, and Shvet Chamni. It has become naturalized in Florida.

The plant is ideal for hydroponic production.

MEDICINAL

CONSTITUENTS- Bacopasaponins (bacoside A & B, bacopaside I, II, bacopasaponin N1, bacopaside III, bacopaside N2), alkaloids such as brahmine and herpestine, D-mannitol, monnierin, bacogenin A1-3, flavonoids luteolin and apigenin, stigmasterol, sitosterol and betulic acid.

Bacopa is widely used in Ayurvedic medicine for epilepsy and asthma, as well as enlarged spleen, anemia, indigestion and inflammation.

The herb is used in Traditional Chinese Medicine, and known as **PA CHI T'IEN**.

The Chinese consider the plant to be slightly warm, pleasant and biting to taste. It helps warm the kidneys and invigorate yang energy.

Therefore, it is widely used for treating impotence, premature ejaculation, "wet dreams", backache, irregular menstruation and cold uterus.

Bacopa is used for "relaxed smartness", with a more even and consistent mood conducive to learning and the expression of ideas and feelings. In fact, it is recommended by numerous herbalists for attention deficit disorder (ADD) and ADHD.

It contains bacosides that should be looked for in our native species, water hyssop.

According to scientists with the Central Drug Research Institute in India, bacosides help to repair damaged neurons by adding muscle to kinase, the protein involved in the synthesis of new neurons. Depleted synaptic activity is thus restored, leading to increased memory capacity. Triterpenoid saponins and their bacosides are believed responsible for enhancing nerve impulse transmission. The latter aid in repairing damaged neurons and restoring synaptic activity.

Bacopa may improve speed of visual information processing, learning rate and consolidation. Stough C et al, *Psychopharmacology* 2001 156:4.

In a double-blind, placebo-controlled, randomized study, the herb shows significant effect on retention of new information. Roodenrys S et al, *Neuropsychopharmacology* 2002 27:2. This study, on adults aged 40-65 years suggests that the herb decreases the rate of forgetting of newly acquired information. Other parameters such as attention, verbal and visual short-term memory, and the retrieval of pre-experimental knowledge were unaffected.

In a study on elderly patients, bacopa enhanced cognitive performance. Calabrese C et al, *The J of Altern Complement Med* 2008 14:6.

Studies are showing promising results for reducing age-related degeneration of vision.

Bacosides, the steroidal saponins in the herb appear to protect neural synapses, especially in the hippocampus, and may have a role to play in Alzheimer's disease.

In one mouse study, it reduced the beta amyloid deposits in brain. Dhanasekaran M et al, *Phytother Res* 2007 21:10.

A systematic review of randomized, controlled human clinical trials found evidence to suggest the herb improves memory free recall. Pase MP et al, *J Altern Compl Med* 2012 18:7 647-52.

A rat memory study of standardized herb found a down regulation of CYP3A suggesting possible interference with drug metabolism and decreased expression of Pgp associated with membrane transport. Singh R et al, *PLoS One* 2013 8:8. Ramasamy S et al, *Molecules* 2014 19(2) also found herb may inhibit P450 enzymes.

A recent study suggests this herb is superior to Gotu Kola (*Centella asiatica*) in anti-oxidant activity. Meena et al, *Ind J Pharmacol* 2012 44:1.

A DB PC crossover study in seventeen normal, healthy participants suggests positive mood effects and reductions in cortisol. Benson S et al, *Phytother Res* 2014 28(4): 551-9.

The plant is considered a febrifuge, nervine and cardiac tonic. It is superior to nux vomica, and considerably less toxic.

Hot poultices are applied to the chest in acute bronchitis, coughs and colds.

The leaf juice, in teaspoon doses, is given to children with catarrh, bronchitis and diarrhea. The leaves are fried and eaten for hoarseness or loss of voice.

The dried leaves are used for debility and low states of exhaustion and nervous breakdown. As an infusion, the leaves help restore blocked urination.

Externally, the leaf juice can be applied to swellings and rheumatic pains.

RECIPES

EXTRACT- standardized to 20% bacosides A & B- 200-400 mg daily in divided doses for average 150 pound adult.

TINCTURE- Produced at 1:2 from fresh plant with 70% alcohol. 5-10 ml daily.

POWDER- 5-10 grams powder.

INFUSION- 8-16 ml daily.

CAUTION- In animal studies, it stimulates T4 activity and may cause elevated thyroid hormone levels. Caution is advised if taking thyroxin, or thyroid suppressing drugs. In this study the T3 levels were not stimulated, but mouse dosages were very high.

THORNY BUFFALOBERRY
(*Shepherdia argentea* [Pursh] Nutt.)
(*Elaeagnus argentea*)
(*E. utilis*)
(*Lepargyrea argentea*)
CANADIAN BUFFALOBERRY
SOAPBERRY
BULL-BERRY
MOOSEBERRY
(*S. canadensis* [L.] Nutt.)
(*L. canadensis*)
(*E. canadensis*)
PARTS USED- berries, winter leaf/twigs

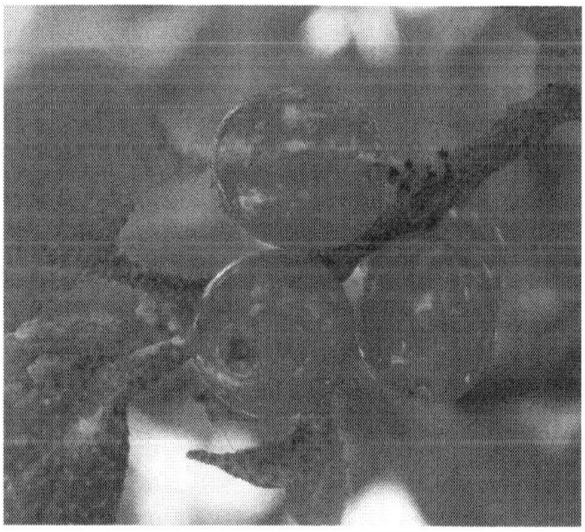

Buffaloberry leaf and fruit

A clump of bull-berry bushes in bloom along the moist edge of a brown pool of freshly melted snow, looks for all the world like a ruffle of time-yellowed lace from grandmother's attic. **A. BROWN**

Shepherdia is named for John Shepherd, an English botanist and horticulturalist of the late 18th and early 19th century. He was curator of the Liverpool Botanical Garden, and the first horticulturist to raise ferns from spores.

Argentea means silver, referring to the silvery, star-shaped hairs on the under leaf. Canadensis means "from Canada". Buffalo berry was name given due to its condiment use as a jelly or sauce with buffalo. Maybe. Bears fatten up on the berries in fall.

Buffaloberry and Soapberry both favor living in open woods, and on dry slopes, near paths, and even gravel soil.

Soapberry (*S. canadensis*) is common to sub-alpine forests and clearings, where you would find fireweed and other earth regenerators. The under side of the leaves have tiny, conspicuous brown scales, or a polka dot appearance. The youngest leaves, at twig tip, look like hands folded in prayer.

The flowers are inconspicuous, yellow green, and appear in early spring and are followed by yellow (rare) to red berries. In most areas, it is a shrub, but can in some areas grow up to eight feet tall.

Shepherdia argentea is much more tree-like (up to 15 feet tall), bearing spines and prefers moister terrain, near rivers and coulees.

The berries contain up to 0.74% saponins. It has brownish flowers, and always an orange red berry.

Various Native tribes used the berries, collecting them by beating the branches over a hide, with a stick. They were then eaten raw, or dried for future use. This is a good way to collect them, as hand picking is tedious, juicy and ineffective.

Preserving was done by placing the ripe berries in a basket, heating with hot rocks, and then spreading them on mats of timber grass to dry. This part of the process was in the open when windy, or near a campfire to speed up the drying. Sometimes the juice from boiling the berries was poured over the drying cakes, a little at a time.

If the berries were dried on grass, they would store them that way. Later, when they whipped them into Indian ice cream, the grass would assist in raising the foam, and the grass would be scooped off the top.

They contain a bitter saponin, that will cause severe blood problems if injected directly into the blood stream, so don't do that.

The Chinook name **SOOPOLALLIE**, comes from soap and berry.

However, upon eating the saponins are converting into steroids and other substances by digestive juices. These saponins make the berries quite soapy and foamy when whipped, hence the name Soapberry. Thorny Buffaloberry can froth, but contains lesser amounts.

Traditionally, the berries were whipped into a dessert called " Indian Ice Cream". When honey or sugar was more readily available, it became the addition of choice.

The Gitksan of northern British Columbia call the treat **YAL IS**. It can be made instantly with ripe berries, the seeds being squeezed out and the juice and a little water whipped by hand into a thick creamy mixture.

Green berries were cooked before whipping, giving a chartreuse-colored foam, while the ripe berries make a delicate pink fluff. Special spoons, carved from caribou ribs, were used for this dessert treat.

Recipes vary throughout our western region, but generally they were boiled overnight in some wooden container with hot rocks, mashed up and spread out to dry on thimbleberry leaves.

The dry cakes were about a quarter inch thick, a foot wide and up to nine feet long.

They use infusions of the dried leaves, picked after berries are ripe, as a diuretic and to treat bladder and uterine infections. The berries are said to increase labor contractions by stimulating the uterus. Leslie Johnson, in her fine doctoral thesis, recorded the whole plant including root as a decoction for chronic coughs, and the root only combined with spruce twigs and needles for rheumatism.

The Dena'ina of Alaska call it **DLIN'A LU** meaning, "mouse's hand", referring to the appearance of the winter buds. They use the stems and branches for tuberculosis, cuts and swellings.

Buffaloberries can be added to stews, or they can be made into jellies, jams, fermented drinks and syrups. The Slave tribe mixed the berries with cooked moose liver or with animal tallow.

The fruit of *S. argentea* is sour, but good raw, while those from *S. canadensis* are insipid and quite bitter. Both berries are improved after first frost.

The berries are rich in iron and vitamin C, but in excess will cause diarrhea, vomiting and cramping of the intestine.

The berry froth can be used as a soap substitute, especially for shampoos; and combines well with horsetail for washing pots and pans during camping trips. The saponin of the berries combines with the silica of horsetail to do a thorough non-polluting job. The berry juice was used as a wilderness type of perm on the hair of pioneer women.

The Woods Cree of Saskatchewan know Soapberry as **KINIPIKOMINANAHTIK** meaning, Snake Berry Tree. It is also called **KINIPIKOMINA**, or Snake Berry Plant. The Cree healer, Russell Willier, calls it Snake Willow, or **KINIPIKNIPSI**. He suggests its use for skin problems, probably due to the saponin content of berries.

The Cree used plant decoctions externally for aching limbs and arthritis. The stem was considered important in the treatment of venereal disease, while the inner bark was infused was a reliable laxative.

The most recent twigs were used in decoction to prevent miscarriage.

A decoction of the fresh, split-peeled roots, and split twigs was given to reduce fever in babies, or used as a rub or rinse for their sore mouths.

The Yukon Athapaskans boil soapberry root or **HOOSHUM**, to help stomach and gall bladder complaints.

Adults as well used the wash for cuts, swellings and skin sores like impetigo.

The root has been added to heart medicines, in an unspecified manner. They are strongly laxative and were used traditionally for chronic coughs and tuberculosis.

The neighboring Gwich'in on the Mackenzie delta call it Mooseberry, or **DINJIK JÀK**. They ate the raw berries for colds or sore throats, and decocted the stems and roots for stomach aches and diarrhea. The roots were sometimes combined with juniper berries and decocted as a laxative, one cup taken before each meal.

The boiled berries were said to increase one's appetite.

Sophie Thomas, native elder and healer from Stoney Creek, B.C. knows the bush as **NUWUSCHUN**. The berries help kill parasites in system, and the stems are decocted and taken internally for cancer.

The branches were decocted as a wash for sore legs, or to soothe mosquito bites and infections that result from scratching. The Dene boiled the berries, often with moose liver or some grease.

For fevers, especially in children, the roots and lower stems were decocted for up to two hours, until the water was red. Two to four ounces were taken at a time.

It would be wise, however, to avoid burning the wood in fires. Some tribes call it Stinkwood, or **MISS-IS-A-MISOI**. Like its close relative, Wolf Willow, the green wood gives off an odour similar to human feces, when burned. Campfire humour.

The Athapaskan tribes used Soapberry decoctions for tuberculosis, and as a wash for cuts and swelling. Be careful with open wounds, as the saponins can be very reactive with blood.

The Wet'suwet'en use **NIWIS** berries for stomach ulcers, while a decoction of the inner bark of branches was used as a laxative or sore stomach.

The Thompson tribe used the stem and leaf decoctions in sweats to help purify them for hunts, or before raiding parties. A leaf and fruit tea is good for ulcers and as a sedative. The branches and leaves were decocted to treat cancer of the stomach and high blood pressure. The neighboring Carrier used the branches in a similar manner. They know the plant as **NUWUS CHUN**.

Decocted soapberry, willow and balsam poplar or cherry bark were used as a poultice wrap for broken bones.

The Secwepemc boiled the twigs and sticks as a laxative tea.

The Navaho ate buffaloberries to help bring down fevers; whereas the Dakota used the fruit in ceremonial feasts at female puberty rites, possibly related to the red colour. The Arapaho name is **AUCH HA HAY BE NA**, the Paiute call it **WEA PU WI**, the Shoshone **WEYUMB**, and the Blackfeet of Montana call it **ME E NIXEN**. The Cheyenne call it **MAT'SI TA SI'MINS**, or red hearted, and collected the berries after the first frost.

The Algonquin, and other tribes used the bark as a medicinal tea.

They used the bark softened in hot water, along with pin cherry bark as a type of plaster cast for broken limbs. When dried, the bark strips would shrink and stiffen, helping hold fractures together. It works, but hawthorn bark is much better if handy.

The Blackfoot name for Thorny Buffaloberry is **MIKSIN-ITSIM**, or Bull berry. The Lakota know it as **MAS'TINCA-PUTE'CAN**, or Rabbit Lip Tree. The Plains Cree name, **MIHKOMINSA** is very similar to the Blackfoot name, and means blood/red berry.

Early voyageurs called it **GRAISSE DE BOEUF**, or Beef Grease, a welcome accompaniment to a monotonous diet of buffalo tongues and steaks.

The Blackfoot would sometimes mash them in a buffalo horn with a stick and drink the juice for stomach problems, or as a mild laxative.

Various British Columbia tribes, including the Nlaka'pamux, Stl'atl'imx and Secwepemc made a type of lemonade from Soapberry juice. This was a refreshing tonic also used for acne, boils, and digestive problems including gallstones.

The saponins were used by hunters, to poison their arrows and spears. If the wild game was not initially killed, they would track it, and it would slowly die from blood hemorrhaging causes by the poison.

Sir John Richardson, known for his search of the Franklin expedition, wrote a book published in 1851. In it, he notes that buffalo berries make a quick and excellent beer that ferments in only 24 hours into a beverage "most agreeable in hot weather".

Mors Kochanski says that the winter leaf tips of buffaloberry are an endorphin inducer, and used by Natives to fend off hunger pains, and other discomforts of winter living. Harmine alkaloids may be responsible, in part, due to their MAO inhibition.

He has observed that the branch buds appear to grow in winter, which is quite unusual.

The nutrient value of *S. canadensis* was studied by Kuhnlein at McGill University in Montreal, and reported *Journal of Food Composition and Analysis* 1989 2.

Buffalo berry is a mercury accumulator, so be careful in polluted regions.

MEDICINAL

CONSTITUENTS- *S. argentea* leaves- caffeic, chlorogenic, coumaric, ferulic, sinapic, gallic, syringic and ellagic acids; isoquercitrin, catechol, tetra-hydroharmol, shephagenins A and B; N,O-diacetyl-tetrahydroharmol, various kaemperferol and querctin rhamnosides.
berries- 12-21% sugars; up to 250 mg% ascorbic acid, beta carotene, leucoanthocyanins, catechols, flavonols.
S. canadensis- root bark- serotonin, shepherdine, tetrahydroharmol.
berries- 1% carotenoid, of which 42% is lycopene, and 45% methyl lycopenate.
Twigs and leaves- harmine, harmaline, harmane, harmol
The root bark of both contains shepherdine, tetrahydroharmol, and N,O-diacetyltetra-hydro-harmol.

Both plants have been poorly studied for medicinal benefit. One study by Ritch-Krc, Turner and Towers at the College of New Caledonia in Prince George, looked at Soapberry, *S. canadensis*. In the *Journal of Ethnopharmacology* 1996 52:3 they reported finding anti-cancer activity against mouse mastocytoma cells in a methanol extract from the stems. The IC50 value was 76 mcg/ml, and indicates a need for further research.

The first author, in her doctoral thesis, found the plant extract activity against *E. coli*, a gram-negative bacterium.

Canadian Buffaloberry is being promoted most actively by Extropian Agroforestry Ventures, Inc. of Lake Alma, Saskatchewan. Over the past ten years, they have planted 100,000 shrubs.

Research indicates leaf, branch and even bark contain compounds able to neutralize 93% of free radicals. According to Morris Johnson, the research director, the plant exhibits, anti-cancer, cardio-protective, anti-viral, and phase 2 enzyme oxidative stress reducer factors.

The berries contain components shown to work with colostrum in maintaining intestinal health.

Saponins froth in water like soap due to half of the molecule being water insoluble. They don't enter our body's cells, but attach themselves to the outside.

Saponins help improve our digestive function, control appetite and regulate what nutrients are absorbed, including glucose. Patients suffering hypoglycemia may benefit, as saponins prevent our pancreas from producing too much insulin.

They inhibit the growth of viruses and aid in regulation of abnormal cell growth, including destruction of cancer cells. Saponins stimulate the immune system by hooking onto receptor sites on immune cells, turbo-charging the immune cell's response.

They help stimulate lymphocyte production, and regulate production of bile. Too little is associated with constipation and inability to metabolize cholesterol, and too much is associated with development of colon cancer and other health issues.

On average, the Japanese eat three times the amount of saponin-rich food as North Americans.

Strong root infusions are used to aid childbirth and were traditionally used for tuberculosis, while berry tinctures are used by midwives to induce parturition.

Berry tinctures benefit the heart, particularly for hypertension, combining well with hawthorn berry.

Thorny buffaloberry (*S. argentea*) was studied for medicinal value, by a team of Japanese researchers led by Yoshida at Okayama University. *Chemical and Pharmaceutical Bulletin* 1996 44:8. They discovered two new hydrolyzable tannins, called Shephagenins A and B, along with hippophaenin A and strictinin.

The tannins show remarkable inhibitory activity against HIV-reverse transcriptase and deserve additional study.

Harmine and Harmol alkaloids decrease cardiac heart rate, myocardial contractile force, and show vasopressin-like effect. Harmaline and related alkaloids induce smooth muscle relaxation, and have therapeutic activity in amoebic dysentery, acting as an anthelmintic. Harmine increases insulin sensitivity and blocks a pathway that normally inhibits fat cells production.

Laboratory studies show rats influenced by harmaline display greater speed in achieving erections and increased frequency of copulation.

Harmine is a reversible MAO inhibitor. It is the same psychoactive compound, banisterine, found in a South American jungle vine, used in the preparation of Ayahuasca. Banisterine was one of the first alkaloids investigated for use in treating Parkinson's disease.

A combination of Reed grass root and buffaloberry tips would be not unlike this infamous psychotropic combination. This is not a recommendation!

Harmine was previously named telepathine, and was used by the Germans in World War II as a truth serum.

Different harmala alkaloids vary in potency. The equivalent of 100 mg harmine is 50 mg harmaline, 35 mg tetrahydryaharman, 25 mg harmalol or harmol, and 4 mg methoxyharmalan. Overdose can cause progressive CNS paralysis.

The berries moderately inhibit aldose reductase, improve glucogen accumulation and reduce expression of both IL-1beta and COX-2.

The berries may provide some protection from diabetic retinopathy and neuropathy via improvement in micro-vascular health and counter metabolic syndrome via improved glucose uptake and energy expenditure. Kraft et al, *J Ag Food Chem* 2008 56:3.

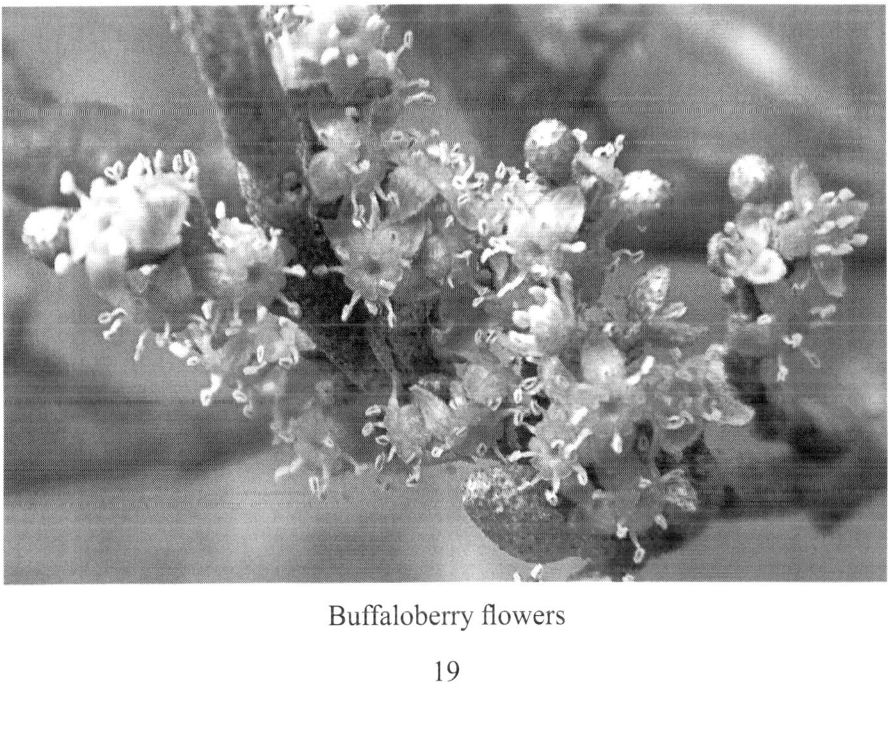

Buffaloberry flowers

FLOWER ESSENCE

Soapberry (*S. canadensis*) essence helps release constrictions around the heart associated with a fear of the power of nature, fear of one's own power, or fear of using one's power in irresponsible, inappropriate and unbalanced ways. **ALASKA**

SPIRITUAL PROPERTIES

There is an Old Blackfoot legend of Old Man, in the days when he had ceased to be a God, and had become a poor, foolish, irrational trickster.

Old Man wandered through the woods one day feeling very hungry.

He came to a deep, still pool and, stooping for a drink, he beheld, lying at the bottom of the pool, a cluster of bright red berries. These were just what he wanted so he tried to reach them by diving after them.

Again and again he dived into the clear water, but could not reach the bottom. Each time he stood on the bank he saw them there in the transparent depths. At last he conceived a plan which could not fail. Tearing strips of bark from trees along the bank, he bound heavy stones about his wrists and neck and waist. Then he dived again.

This time, he reached the bottom- but there were not berries there. When he decided to return to the surface, however, the stones still held him to the bottom, head down, feet floating far above. He had a desperate struggle to unloose the strings of bark, but at last he threw himself half-drowned on the soft bank of the pond.

As he lay there, gasping and choking for air, he looked up into the tangled branches above and there, scarcely higher than his own head, was the cluster of berries he had been diving after. Furious at being so deceived, he seized a stick and beat the bushes until the branches were broken and the berries dropped to the ground. "Your branches will always look broken and people will always gather your berries by beating you", he told the tree. And people always have.

ANNORA BROWN

In a Bella Coola myth, the origin of soapberries is described. Raven was invited to a feast by a certain mountain in the interior of British Columbia, which as a chief with human traits.

Soapberries were abundant on his slopes, but he only wanted to keep them for his guests. Raven was inside the mountain with other animals and birds, but all the entrances were closed.

Raven used his power to make one of the guests go outside, and as soon as the entrance opened, he seized a soapberry branch and flew away, dropping some berries as he went.

Wherever the berries dropped, new plants grew, and from then on the Bella Coola could make Indian Ice Cream whenever they wanted.

McILWRAITH

PERSONALITY TRAITS

Holy Man saw a group of buffalo, and followed them a long way, until they revealed themselves as Buffalo people. They taught him painting, and prayers, and gave him two women as wives. He has sex with the buffalo women, and he became ill, but was healed by herbs.

The Buffalo women were wives of the great Buffalo Who Never Dies. He came to avenge this indignity.

Holy Man and the two wives escaped to the mountains. Each time Buffalo Who Never Dies charged the mountains, a part of them was demolished. Holy Man kept moving, and then put an arrow into his adversary.

On the fourth charge, the arrows took effect and Buffalo rolled over and died. Since he embodied the life of all the Buffalo people, they all died expect the two wives of Holy Man. With their encouragement, he set about restoring the great Buffalo to life. He pulled out the arrows with ceremony and prayer.

Finally Buffalo Who Never Dies began to move, and when completely restored, he recognized Holy Man's superior power and all claim to his wives. Holy Man stayed with the Buffalo People, for some time, learning their lore. Then he made his way back to those waiting for him at Whirling Mountain.

NAVAHO LEGEND

RECIPES

BERRY TINCTURE- 1:3 at 50% fresh berries. One teaspoon as needed.

BUFFALO BERRY JELLY- Wash and stem one quart of ripe berries, place in saucepan and add one half cup of cold water. Bring to boil and simmer for 10 minutes. Crush berries and simmer for five more minutes. Run through a food mill, and jelly bag.

Measure fruit juice, and add 1.5 cups for each cup of juice. Mix well and bring to boil. Add three ounces of pectin and boil for one full minute. Stir constantly. Skim off foam, and pour into sterilized jars.

Note: If berries are picked before frost, pectin is not needed.

BUFFALO BERRY CONSERVE- Wash and clean 4 cups of berries. Add to saucepan with one and a half cups of water. Cook until soft. Add four ounces of chopped currants, one half cup of chopped hazelnuts, one chopped orange and 8 cups of sugar. Mix and stir constantly for 20 minutes. Skim off foam and pour into sterilized jars.

INDIAN ICE CREAM- Add one-quarter cup to each quart of fresh berries, or two tablespoons of dried berries. Beat the mixture into light foam, until the consistency of egg whites. You can add some sugar as the foam is forming if you like (3-4 tbsp. per cup of berries). Traditionally, saskatoons and other berries were added as sweeteners.

Green soapberries make white foam, the ripe berries a pink or salmon colour. Do not allow any grease or oil to contact the berries or they won't whip up.

DANDRUFF SHAMPOO and CONDITIONER- Combine equal parts of dried buffalo berries and dogwood berries in water and decoct for ten minutes. Allow to stand until cool, strain, and use immediately or store in fridge.

CAUTION- Do not take ingest leaf extracts with prescription drugs of any kind.

CALAMUS ROOT
SWEET FLAG
MUSKRAT ROOT
(*Acorus americanus* [Raf.] Raf**)**
(*A. calamus auct.non* L.**)**
(*A. odoratus*)
(*A. aromaticus*)
PARTS USED- root and leaves

It was the tall, sweet-scented Flag,
Lay pictured there so true,
I could have deem'd some Fairy hand
The faithful image drew.
The falchion-leaves, all long and sharp;
The stem, like a tall leaf too,
Except where, half-way up its side,
A cone-shaped flower-spike grew... **TWAMLEY**

The flower is a long thing...of a greenish yellow color, curiously checkered, as if it were wrought with a needle with green and yellow silk intermixt. **GERARD**

You are often more bitter than I can bear,
You burn and sting me,
Yet you are beautiful to me your faint tinged roots.
WALT WHITMAN

Calamus is from the Greek **KALAMOS** or Arabic **KALON** meaning pen or reed, and originally from the Sanskrit **KALAMAS**. Kalamos was the son of the river god Maeander, who loved Karpos, the son of Zephyrus and Chloris. When Karpos drowned, Kalamos was transformed into a reed, whose rustling song is a sigh of lamentation. Vacha is the Sanskrit name for the plant meaning "power of the voice".

Calamari, meaning squid from the Latin **CALAMARIUM**, "ink horn" or "pen case"; Calumet, another name for a Native Peace Pipe made from the hollow reed, and Chalumeau, the lower notes of a clarinet's range, are all related words.

Acorus is from the Greek or Arabic **AKORON** from **KORE** or **COREON** for pupil of the eye. Andrzej Szczeklik writes. "The Greeks placed the soul elsewhere. They imagined it in the form of a little doll, visible through the pupil of the eye, which as a result they called the kore." Kore is another name for Persephone, the Greek goddess.

This reedy, water plant is familiar to ponds, sloughs and permanently wet ground throughout the prairies.

At first glance it appears like a cattail; but on closer inspection it's true nature is revealed. Albertazzi et al, *Molecular and General Genetics* 1998 259:6 suggests that Sweet Flag might be the most ancient surviving representative of the ancestral monocotyledonous plants.

The plant is placed under the Moon, due to its half moon shape, watery nature and yellow colour of the inflorescence.

The plants have been prized and praised throughout the world; and we are most fortunate that the safest variety is our western North American asarone-free diploid (2n=24) type. This plant produces viable seed and was probably chosen for planting across western North America. It has 2-6 raised veins and a swollen centre to the leaf in cross section.

In China, the Moso sorcerers have used sweet flag in rituals for over 2000 years. During the 11th century, the Tatars moved sweet flag from India to Russia and Poland. They believed the plant purified drinking water, and so they carried and planted it in their new settlements.

Traditional Chinese Medicine uses calamus root, **SHIH CHANG PU**, to treat deafness, dizziness, and epilepsy. Other names include **PAI CH'ANG-P'U**, white calamus, and **CHIEN CH'ANG-P'U**, sword calamus.

It is highly prized for the ability to restore speech after a stroke. Studies from China show its value in lowering blood pressure, clearing lungs, and killing bacteria. The leaves of sweet flag and mugwort are used as a charm during the dragon boat festival, and on the 5th day of the 5th month, the leaves are hung on doors to ward off evil spirits.

Remains of sweet flag have been found in the tomb of King Tut. Several Egyptian perfume and unguent recipes contain the fragrant calamus root, including the famous kyphi. Hebrew tradition pressed oil from the roots for application in the Tabernacle.

Mongolian traditional medicine uses tea and tincture as a tonic, appetizer, and to treat stomachache, intestinal disorders, and some skin diseases. It is used as a snuff powder in Tibet.

In Japan, the plant symbolizes a Samurai's bravery, due to the sword like leaves. On May 5th, during the Boy's Festival (Tango no Sekku), many families enjoy the Sweet Flag Bath or Shobu Yu.

In India, the related *A. angustatus* is promoted as an herb that improves mental focus, and reduces epileptic seizures. The root, combined with cardamom, helps the digestion of dairy products. In Ayurvedic medicine, the herb is known as **PUVACHA**.

Vacha means literally "speak" and is descriptive of the self-expression or intelligence stimulated by the plant. It is found in Indian and Tibetan incense mixtures for its illuminating and strengthening effect on the mind, strengthening of nerves and increase of meditative powers. According to Lad and Frawley it is "nourishment for the Kundalini serpent". It relieves anxiety, and may be worth trying in cases of OCD, or obsessive-compulsive disorder.

The Arabian physician Ibn Al-Baitar, in his *Collection of Simple Remedies* (ca 1225 BC), recommended Calamus as it "warms up blood and is useful for cold temperaments".

Calamus was widely prized for warding off the black plague, and its use in a variety of contagious disease can be traced back to Byzantine medicine.

The Old English Herbarium translated into Anglo-Saxon over a millennium ago, recommended Calamus root simmered down to two thirds in water and given for three days to those that cannot urinate.

During the Crimean War of 1854, the allied French and British armies were recommended to take calamus root against marsh pestilence, as quinine was in short supply.

Cathedrals and other places of worship throughout the world have strewn the leaves on the floor in order to scent and purify. The leaves have a smell mildly like tangerine peel, with a vanilla undertone.

It is much mentioned in the Bible, and was immortalized by the mystic poet, Walt Whitman, in his famous *Leaves of Grass*.

Forty-five ballads under the Calamus chapter were symbolic of the love of male comrades, adhesiveness and personal attachment. Calamus has long symbolized male love, perhaps due in part, to the symbolic penis-like spathe.

The leaf buds are a good edible as are the flowers. Children of Holland chew the root like a gum.

In Lithuania, the rhizome is soaked in brandy, and used for chest pains and diarrhea. The leaves are added to hot baths to relieve pain, gout and rheumatism.

Indeed, the root is a good ginger or cinnamon substitute in many recipes. Candied roots, made by boiling sliced roots in maple syrup, are just like ginger in taste and use. Benedictine and Chartreuse liqueurs, various beers, Vermouth de Turin and gin all use calamus oil for flavouring at rates from 10-30 ppm. The root was a one time used to flavour beer and give it a clear appearance. For schnapps and other liqueurs produced in Germany, the asarone content cannot exceed one mg/litre. Stockton Bitters, a tonic medicine from England, contains calamus and gentian root.

The leaves were used as a base for baking bread throughout Eastern Europe. The inner stem was widely eaten.

The leaves make a great seasoning in fish soups and stews. Calamus root and mint leaves make interesting vinegar, as does the leaf essential oil.

The root powder has been substituted for orrisroot as a fixative in tooth and hair powders, dry shampoos; as well as the French snuff a la violette.

The Cree of Northern Alberta make great use of this muskrat food, known as **WACHASKOMECHIWIN**.

It is also known as rat root or muskrat root, **WACASKWATAPIH**, or simply **WIHKES** or **WIYIKIYO**. The Eastern Ojibwa name is very similar, **WIKE**, or **WEE-KEES**.

Cree around Hudson Bay, call it fire or bitter pepper root, or **POW E MEN ARTIC**.

The Chipewyan also call it muskrat food, or **DZEN NI**. Muskrat is a traditionally favourite food of many northern tribes. The muskrat feeds heavily on calamus, and its rich, dark winter meat is so highly scented, it is said eating the cooked meat is like ingesting a valuable medicine. I find myself humming the song Muskrat Love, while gathering the root in late summer at the annual Rat Root Rendezvous west of Edmonton.

The root is gathered and used for colds, headaches, and other stomach complaints. The weekend is also a good excuse for wilderness and survival guides, wildcrafters and others to get together for a casual weekend.

The root is slowly chewed and used to overcome fatigue on long journeys.

It cuts phlegm and is used in relieving asthma. For cramped arms and legs, paralyzed limbs or rheumatic swellings, poultices or hot fomentations are applied to affected areas.

It is often chewed for diabetes, or held in the throat for a long time to "get rid of the tonsils by burning them off."

For earache, a small piece of root is softened in water and inserted in ear. Not too far in!

The Dene smudge dried rat root and inhale the smoke for headaches. The crushed root is boiled and cooled for stomachache and to help pass pinworms. Some Dogrib or Dene healers say that rat root should not be taken within a few hours of modern medicines.

Native drummers will often tie a string on the root and hang it around their neck. They can then chew and suck on it to keep their singing voices strong hour after hour, hence the name Drummer's or Singer's root. The dried root resembles the trachea, in the doctrine of signatures.

The Blood, like Eastern Cree call it **POW-E-MEN-ARTIC** or fire root, and used it to relieve coughs and treat liver ailments. The Blackfoot had to trade for the root and used it with tobacco as a smoking mixture, or alone as an abortifacient.

The Sioux and Dakota chewed calamus root and rubbed the paste on their faces to prevent excitement and fear.

Others mixed oil with the burnt root for flatulence and colic.

The roots are said to yield a mildly hallucinogenic property if taken in excess. Two inches of the root is medicinal; while eight is considered bordering on an unknown journey. I have never found that to be the case personally. This is based on the beta asarone rich root found elsewhere, I believe.

On the Sisseton Indian reservation in South Dakota, rat root and another unspecified root are boiled together as a tea to take the place of insulin, or simply chewed to treat high blood sugar levels.

The Chippewa combined roots of wild sarsaparilla (*Aralia nudicaulis*) and calamus in decoction for soaking their fishing nets. Another combination was calamus root, prickly ash bark, sassafras, and wild ginger root for colds and bronchitis.

Chippewa used the root as a mordant with bloodroot for dyeing.

Various tribes, including the Omaha and Sioux used the root powder, or infusions for their horses as a race stimulant; and made aromatic garlands of the leaves. The Omaha and Ponca name is **MAKAN NINIDA**, while the Osage name **PEXE BOAO'KA**, means flat herb.

John Lame Deer, a Lakota healer had this to say. "**SINKPE TAWOTE**- that's muskrat food, sweet flag, one of our busiest medicines. It has bitter roots that are very good against a fever. When you grind them up and mix them with gunpowder they are a help against cramps in the arms and legs."

The Iroquois used the root in a variety of ways and in different combination. The powdered root in hot infusion for colds and chills, the powdered root in cold water for indigestion.

The root was combined with water milfoil for slow circulation in adolescents, with plantain root for painful breathing, and with arrowhead root for night crying by babies and young children.

The Algonquin combined the root tea with chokecherry bark for coughs. The Ojibwa used the root medicinally and call it

POWEMENARCTIC, or muskrat root. Note the extreme similarity to the Blood name.

The Cheyenne call it bitter medicine, or **WI'UKH IS E'EVO**, and traded with their Sioux neighbors for the root. They tied a small piece on their children's necklace for both protection from night spirits and for numbing teething pain. They also tossed pieces of the root on glowing rocks in the sweat lodge for cleansing purpose. The powdered root was combined with bark of red osier dogwood in smoking mixtures.

It was known as a "ghost medicine" with the power to ward off evil.

The leaves were also braided or added to baby bundles for good luck and as an aromatic insecticide. The innermost tender leaf is edible as is the flower bud before flowering.

The Pawnee name is **KAIITSHA ITU**, meaning "medicine lying in water". The young green blades were braided into fragrant neck garlands.

The Lakota name **SINKE TAWOTE** means "muskrat food". The specific name for the root **SUNKACE** meaning, "dog penis" refers to the phallic shape of the flower.

Ayurvedic physicians use calamus root as a specific for schizophrenia.

In Brazil, the root is considered anthelmintic, while in neighboring Argentina, the root is given to relieve painful menstruation.

Nine worldwide plant patents exist, including shampoo, toothpaste, liqueurs, and treating diarrhea and flatulence in farm animals.

The dried powder can be used with birds to get rid of lice, killing them off in 12 hours. The root infusion is used in India to wash newborn calves for protection against insects and disease.

When the root is very dry, you can ignite one end, and breath the smoke for headaches, and stuffy colds.

Work by one student of Dr. Robin Marles showed that straight linear cuts through patches for wild crafted calamus root is the most efficacious for regeneration, versus the clearcut approach. Commercial planting will produce over a ton of root per acre.

Several authors have mentioned that mosquitoes are not found in water where calamus is found. I believe they are right!

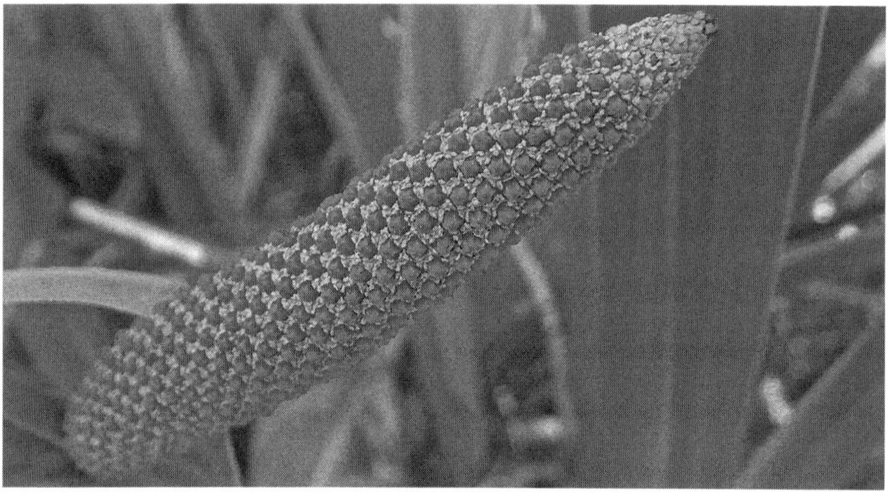

Calamus root seedhead

MEDICINAL

CONSTITUENTS- root- 243 components including mainly sesquiterpene and monoterpenes ketones, acorone 5246 ppm, aconic and acoric acid, mucilage, bitters, tannins, choline, essential oils, acorin, acoretin, galangin, furfural, shyobunone and iso-shyobunone.
Also includes 6-epishyobunone, 2,6-diepishyobunone, acorafuran, acorone, acoragermacrone, isoacoranone, and acorenone, geranylacetate, and small amounts of calamendiols.
Beta asarone (cis-isoasarone) may or may not be present in diploid type; and if so at extremely low percentage. Alpha asarone may be present in low amounts, and amines, such as dimethyl-amine, methyl amine, trimethylamine as well as choline are also present.
plant- tropone, beta curcumene, acolamone, acoragermacrone, acoric acid, acorine, ascorbic acid, borneol, calarene, delta-guazulene, dimethylamine, mycrene, saponins, tannins, trans anethole, trimethylamine.

Calamus root is used, as a cold infusion, for all manner of digestive complaints, including hyperacidity. It stimulates the salivary glands, and yet counteracts acidity and reduces heartburn and gas; combining well with meadowsweet or queen of the meadow.

Cold infusions of the root help pancreatic function, one sip before and one sip after meals three times daily, in cases of mild late onset diabetes.

It is highly prized for its specific action on stomach cancer, working in a similar manner to condurango vine of South America.

In Europe, our calamus root is much prized for this purpose, and warrants further investigation.

Small pieces can be chewed for helping kick addiction such as nicotine.

When chewed, the juice released causes nausea and works as an aversion therapy. It also affects the brain during withdrawal from cocaine, marijuana, heroin and morphine. During this time, addicts experience intense craving, nausea and vomiting, that acorus can help modify. Later, when the brain can be stimulated by wheat, meat and milk, acorus seems to enable the process by which the brain recognizes these non-drug opiates.

The herbalist 7Song suggests chewing the root is good for a pot hangover. Matthew Wood writes of cases where it appears palliative in Alzheimer's disease.

Small pieces of dried root relieve toothache and teething pain in young children.

Tincture of the fresh root is a good parasiticide applied to the skin for treating lice, scabies and crabs. The root is powdered and rubbed into affected areas. A hot poultice of the mashed or powdered root can be applied to injured extremities where circulation is impaired and tissue damage severe.

It is most useful in metabolic sluggishness, where there is an accumulation of toxins. Like Bogbean, it is a gentle, cleansing herb. Calamus root is good for digestive stagnation, associated with gas, bloating, eructation and congestion.

A body temperature enema can be helpful in rectal pains associated with hemorrhoids, bleeding or inflammation. Be careful with irritable bowel, as the root is not demulcent.

Individuals with low grade annoying fevers, and poor vital energy will like this herb. Choline counteracts excessive cholesterol and the manner in which arteries handle its potential buildup.

Sweet flag helps promote menses delayed by chilled or exhausted dispositions. Decoctions are useful in muscle spasms, restlessness and insomnia, as well as sedative to the central nervous system. Acoric acid is a sesquiterpene with hypotensive properties. Other authors have speculated that the high levels of organic potassium help relieve asthma, hay fever, hiccups and even muscular dystrophy. This is too simple an explanation.

The asarone-free genotype of calamus showed anti-spasmodic properties on par with standard antihistamines, in a study by Keller et al *Planta Medica* 1985 1 6-9. Other calamus genotypes do not have this property. Work by Gilani et al, *Phyto Res* 2006 20:12 confirmed this anti-spasmodic nature and suggested the activity was calcium channel-like in nature. It has shown to be anti-fungal and anti-bacterial, but not anti-viral.

Scientists have identified other compounds in acorus that act on the body chemicals other than histamine, to stop bronchial constriction during asthmatic attacks.

Methyl isoeugenol, for example is an expectorant, anti-spasmodic, anti-histaminic and anti-bacterial. Shah et al, *J Ethnopharm* 131:2 determined broncho-dilating activity.

It makes a stimulating morning bath; showing the different effect gained by external vs. internal application. Baths are very useful for general exhaustion during convalescence, anemia and diabetic conditions.

Gary Raven, a traditional healer from Manitoba, recommends calamus, wild licorice and white water lily root be grated and used as a tea to treat diabetes. Small slices can be chewed to treat high cholesterol. Work by Parab and Mengi, *Fitoterapia* 2002 73:6 on the Indian variety showed significant hypolipidemic activity.

Rau et al, *Pharmazie* 2006 61:11 found calamus root very active on the human peroxisome proliferator-activated receptor associated with fat and blood sugar regulation.

Other herbs showing similar activity include corn silk, cayenne, water plantain and stinging nettle.

Work by Acuna et al, on our North American calamus, found high anti-oxidant activity in ethanol extracts of the rhizome. *Phytother Res* 2002 16:1.

A substance other than beta-asarone in calamus root, extracted by ethyl acetate, enhances adipocyte differentiation and may have benefit the treatment of type 2 diabetic conditions. It appears to have a rosiglitazone-like activity. Wu et al, *Phytother Res* 21:6.

Calamus root appears to decrease serum glucose and triglycerides, and increase insulin sensitivity in genetically obese mice. Wu et al, *J Ethnopharm* 2009 123:2.

Tis Mal Crow, a Native American root doctor, uses Calamus root as an activator or accelerator that increases the potency of other herbs. He believes it should only be added in one part to 32 parts of other herbs, or the mixture may be dangerously strong. Calamus is used specifically with white flowered medicines for this purpose; violet leaves for green medicines.

Calamus root protects brain tissue from free radicals produced by excessive oxygen. This can occur in various brain related disorders, including stroke, where a restored flow of oxygen to previously deprived cells can cause brain tissue damage. A formula of calamus root and Oriental Cedar seed (*Thuja orientalis*), as well as Figwort, Lycium fruit and Licorice root is used in TCM for ADD, depression and Alzheimer's disease.

It may be useful in preventing epileptic activity. Hazra et al, *Human Exp Toxicol* 2007 26:12.

Acorus root lectins have been identified by Bains et al, *Int Immunopharm* 2005 5:9 and show significant inhibition of J774, a murine macrophage cancer cell line, and to a lesser extent a B cell lymphoma. Shulka et al, *Phytother Res* 2002 16 found *Acorus calamus* protects against acrylamide-induced neuro-toxicity.

High fat, fried foods such as french fries and charred meat create acrylamides. Chew a piece of the root before or after a poutine or barbecue indulgence.

Work by Parab et al, *Fitoterapia* 2002 73:6 found saponins and ethanol extracts in the root demonstrate significant hypolipidemic activity.

Mehorotra et al, *Int Immunopharm* 2003 3:1 found calamus root extracts demonstrate both anti-proliferative and immuno-suppressive potential *in vitro*.

The leaves of *A. calamus* inhibit pro-inflammatory cytokine release and may be useful for treating skin disease. Kim et al, *J Ethnopharm* 2009 122:1.

TMA-2, a controlled drug in the United States, is a hallucinogen with at least ten times the potency of mescaline. Asarone is naturally converted to TMA-2 in the body by amination shortly after ingestion. This only occurs when either alpha or beta asarone is present, however. In chemical structure alpha asarone is similar to mescaline, from the peyote cactus, while beta asarone is more chemically like myristicin and compounds in kava kava. The wild, western North American root contains little of either asarone. It appears that European roots have been planted and are taking hold in the northeastern United States. This introduced cytotype does contain asarone derivatives.

Beta asarone may be of benefit in cognitive impairment including Alzheimer's disease. Geng et al, *Biol Pharm Bull* 2010 33:5. It is also toxic.

ESSENTIAL OIL

CONSTITUENTS- *A. americanus-* shyobunone, isoshyobunone (8-13%), beta-farnesene, methyl eugenol, calamenen (4%), beta sesquiphellandrene (3%), pre-isocalamenediol (7%), calamenol (5%), cadinol, linalool, calamone, azulene, camphor, acolamone, pinene, acorone (11%), acorenone (0-18%), asaraldehyde and cineole among 243 recorded volatile components. Up to 26% acorone may also be present in dried roots. The aldehyde with characteristic odour is (Z, Z)-4,7-decadienal ($C_{10}H_{16}O$). Its concentration in the oil is 500 ppm, and the odour threshold value 4.2 ppb.

The concentration is about 100,000 times its odour threshold, indicating the importance of this compound to overall odour composition.

Steam distillation of the fresh root yields a reddish volatile oil (up to 6%) that is heavy, earthy, and slightly sweet with bitter undertones. It is described by some writers as resembling dried milk and sweet leather, and compared to the fragrance of a milk-truck or a shoe repair shop by authors like Arctander.

The oil from fresh rhizomes is finer and more soluble in weak alcohol. In my own distillations, at 40% moisture, the yield is about 0.7%. The fresh rhizome oil of asarone-free calamus is very difficult to find on the world market and definitely has a demand.

The outer rhizome peel contains the most essential oil, and should not be peeled for distillation.

Oil from the leaves is a straw yellow camphorous product containing butyric and oenanthylic acids as esters. Yield is about 0.5-1% from leaves.

Calamus oil was used by the Egyptians in ointment given to Moses that also contained myrrh, cinnamon, and cassia in olive oil.

Its mind-altering effects are used for meditation and psychic development and in perfume blends for smooth middle notes. The North American fragrance market presently uses over $30 million of imported oils annually.

Beta-asarone is low or undetectable in the diploid cytotype North American oil. Keller et al, *Planta Medica* 1983 47:2.

It can be used for congested kidneys and bladder infections. Bronchitis and asthmatic complaints where there is need for anti-bacterial and anti-spasmodic properties suggests using calamus oil

Isoasarone free oil from Canadian calamus exhibits anti-spasmodic effect, while oils from Indian Calamus, containing up to 96% isoasarone, have no spasmolytic effect.

The essential oil of diploid calamus has anti-spasmodic action not found in the other varieties, according to studies by Locock, *Can Pharm Journal* 1987 120.

Either steam or rub the oil in a vegetable oil into the chest to achieve this calming effect. Massages relax tense and sore muscles; tired feet and varicose veins feel rejuvenated and toned. For a footbath use calamus oil and a dispersant in hot water or a few drops of oil in a hot bath to relieve menopausal hot flashes.

Although no studies have been conducted on the olfactory effect of our native diploid essential oil, work by Koo et al, *Biol Pharm Bull* 2003 26:7 looked at the effect of fragrance inhalation of *A. gramineus* root essential oil. Significant sedative and anti-convulsant effect was noted, and increased GABA levels in the brain.

The scent prolonged sleeping time in a dose dependent manner. Studies on our native species would be useful.

Calamus oil is mixed in silverweed tincture as a mouthwash for gingivitis.

It is a digestive and biliary stimulant, useful in anorexia, gas pains and digestive spasms. The oil clears phlegm in the gastrointestinal tract and calms nervous problems such as vertigo and tension headaches. The oil will also assist those with intermittent fevers, and is mildly vermifuge in action.

It has been noted that considerable amounts of heat are given off at the time of flowering. Perhaps the flowers could be experimentally distilled and investigated further.

Studies in the Czech Republic found that the essential oil content was higher in the spring (0.8-2.6%), than in the fall (1.0-1.8%). Although it may not be relevant to North America, the same researchers found a close negative relationship between essential oil content and the concentration of calcium in the water and the pH of the substrate.

Work by Stahl et al, *Planta Med* 47:2 found CO_2 extraction retained more of the bitter and sesquiterpene components.

Work in Russia found rhizomes and roots dried in the sun yielded 10% and 30% less essential oil respectively than plant material dried in the shade.

Calamus root oil is often combined with catnip oil, and beaver castor as a muskrat lure.

Work by Bertea et al, *Phytochemistry* 2005 66:5 developed a good sequence analysis to distinguish the diploid type from other.

This would be useful to industry and government in helping our native root take its rightful place as a useful medicinal herb.

The supercritical carbon dioxide extraction yields oil containing acorone and isoacorone (37%) acoragermacrone (12%) acorenone (6%) and shyobunone isomers (2%). Acoragermacrone usually degrades to shyobunone in steam distillation.

HYDROSOL

The hydrosol of dried Canadian calamus root is masculine and earthy, while the fresh root is similar but even greener. I like both, but many people find it too intense. The pH is 4.6.

Suzanne Catty says, in her excellent book says "the hydrosol makes a gently astringent aftershave on its own or combined with sandalwood, cedar wood or bay laurel.

It probably has some benefit in various digestive problems concerning the liver, stomach and pancreas, and is worthy of further research."

PLANT OILS

Calamus stems contain lipid fractions composed of 64.5% neutral lipids, 28% glyco-lipids, and 7.3% phospholipids.

The root contains similar phospholipids, but 11% more neutral lipids and similar drop in glyco-lipid content.

Palmitic acid predominates both glyco- and phospholipid content, while linolenic acid predominates in the leaves and stems. Yield of total lipids in leaf is about 2.9%

Palmitoleinic acid is concentrated mainly in the neutral fraction of the root. Total root lipids are 5.6%.

FLOWER ESSENCES

The plant signature of calamus is somewhat complex and esoteric, breaking down into threes and sixes. These numbers are associated with the mind, body and spirit-which the flower essence treats. There is a remarkable resemblance between the human aura, and the stamen and ovaries of the plant.

The flower essence integrates by merging the mental, emotional and etheric bodies.

This activity makes Sweet Flag an enhancer of other flower essences, and especially useful in schizophrenia.

Consider this essence for extremes of anxiety, stress, or fear; especially if the issues involve death. Practitioners in the hospice movement would benefit from the use of this essence. It physically stimulates capillary action by penetrating the ductless gland system.

Make use of the essence for preparing animals for stress, like car rides and new homes. Plants being transplanted would benefit from watering containing the calamus flower essence. **GURUDAS**

Sweet Flag flower essence brings you strength for new beginnings. It affects the brow and the heart and helps to unravel cross energies that cause a buildup above the throat and the abdomen. **OLIVE**

Calamus flower essence is helpful to those individuals who have difficulty with temperature regulation. Cold or hot night sweats, menopausal flushes; or individuals who experience one-sided heat or cold in body would benefit.

Also, individuals who have noticeable heat loss from the head, or who are sulphur types homeopathically, may find this flower essence especially useful. **PRAIRIE DEVA**

MYTHS AND LEGENDS

It is said that in the old days, the Penobscot people were suffering from a great plague. Many were ill, many had died. One of the leaders, severely troubled about the illness sweeping his people, prayed to the Creator for help. That night, the Muskrat appeared to him in his dreams.

"You have prayed for help for your people", said the Muskrat, " and I have come to help you. Look carefully and remember."

The man looked closely and saw the Muskrat turn himself into a plant. He examined the plant closely until he knew it well. He looked deeper and saw that the spirit and power of the Muskrat was contained within the root of the plant and thus knew that this was the part of the plant he was to use.

When he awoke, he dressed and traveled to the place where he had been shown the plant would be found. There he dug it up and made medicine for his people. In this way the Penobscot people were healed and sweet flag, muskrat root came to the people.

PENOBSCOT TALE

SPIRITUAL PROPERTIES

Kore is the Ancient Greek word for a girl, and also for the pupil of the eye. The Greeks said that the soul was visible in the form of a little girl, through the pupil. How could they have know that the pupil is the one and only tiny window that gives a view of the brain and of the ocular nerves? **ANDRZEJ SZCZEKLIK**

If you find yourself worrying about your finances, cut up the dried roots and place them in the corners of the rooms of your house to ensure yourself of always having more than enough money. The dried root can be used in incense to encourage spiritual, emotional and physical healing. **S. GREGG**

PERSONALITY TRAITS

Calamus is another good doctrine of signatures plant. It grows in the swamp or bog in really smelly and sulfurous places, the coldest, dankest part of the swamp. The root also looks like a larynx. This shows us that it is good for colds and congestion, breaks up phlegm, and is good for the throat and voice. **TIS MAL CROW**

Sweet flag is generally considered a stomach tonic and appetite increaser. Many time addicted patients have to go through a waking up period, realizing the ramifications of what they have been living and to begin to change their minds. Sweet flag is gentle in its action and seems to really help bring about a change of consciousness. It will help bring about a stronger sense of resolve for the patient and their decision to change things. **K. PROEFROCK ND**

A woman in her fifties fell down a mountainside and sustained a head injury. She was extremely debilitated, to the point where she would get lost for hours two blocks from home. We tried peony root without success and then Calamus.

She said the effect was immediate, profound, and highly beneficial. Each time she took the tincture, the plant seemed to say to her "Concentrate." It taught her a new and different way of thinking and rescued her from an almost helpless state. **WOOD**

BOTANICA POETICA

Calamus to calm you down
A G. I. tonic quite renown
If colic is the situation
Spasm or nervous tension
Relax and soothe, it's known to do
A G. I. cramp it will undo
Volatile oils there are within
Reducing flatulence therein
Ulcer, gastritis, a poor appetite
Sweet Flag helps to set things right
A demulcent to coat and soothe
Dyspepsia you could improve
It's a spice that clears the mind
Better focus you will find
To quit tobacco, ease the hype
For the excited nervous type
But here's a piece a sound advice
Don't abuse this bitter spice
Not high dose, not continuous
Otherwise it's dangerous
So when you think of Calamus
Think aromatic bitter, par excellence!

SYLVIA CHATROUX

RECIPES

COLD INFUSION- This is necessary as heat and boiling destroy some vital properties. Soak one ounce of chopped fresh or dried root in a pint of water overnight. Gently warm in morning and use one half cup before meals.

TINCTURE- twenty to thirty drops up to three times daily. Small amounts reduce stomach acidity, while larger doses increase acid production. Make a fresh root tincture at 70% at 1:2, or from the dried at 1:4 and 50% alcohol.

ESSENTIAL OIL- 2-3 drops twice daily. If used externally, dilute with carrier oil. It works like arnica for relieving deep pain. Do not use during pregnancy.

DECOCTION- for bath- Bring one ounce of root to simmer in one quart of water. Simmer twenty minutes. Strain and add to a hot bath for nervous exhaustion.

For enema, use only 2 tsp of dried root to 150 ml of water. Strain and cool to body temperature. Work by Chen et al, *Planta Medica* 2009 June 8 found a one hour decoction reduced beta asarone in European roots by 85%.

CAUTION- Avoid during pregnancy. It is worthy of note, that the European calamus, that contains up to 15% beta-asarone is considered free of side effects or health hazards, by the *PDR for Herbal Medicines*, when taken in therapeutic doses.

There is considerable confusion over the viability of *A. americanus* seeds. I have never been able to germinate seeds from northern Alberta, but numerous authors cite the species seeds are fertile. My friend Gordon Steinrath assures me the seeds DO germinate.

The original studies by Taylor, Gross et al, *Tox Appl Pharm* 1967 10 405 fed rats a diet containing 5000 ppm of Asian calamus oil, until they formed malignant intestinal tumors. So what?

CANBY'S LOVAGE

(*Ligusticum canbyi* J. M Coult & Rose**)**
PARTS USED- root

Lovage derives from love-ache, meaning love parsley in an early translation from Old French to Middle English. Ligusticum is from the Greek for a related plant used by Dioscorides. Perhaps, obscurely, of Liguria, Italy, where the medicinal Lovage was first described.

Canbyi is named for William Canby, a 19th century businessman from Delaware, who enjoyed adding new plants to his extensive herbarium collection.

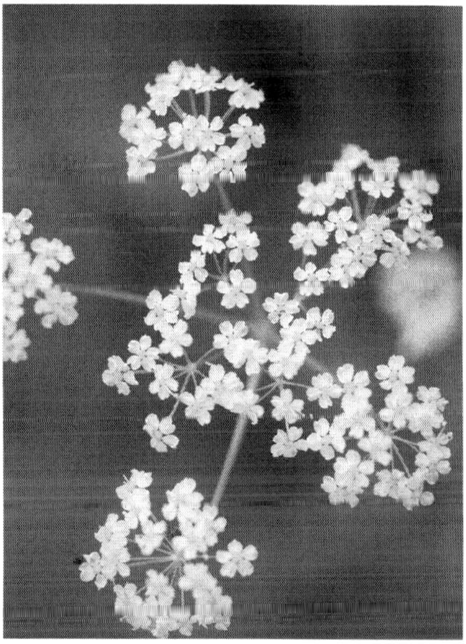

Osha flowers in full bloom

Canby's Lovage has not been found on this side of the continental divide in Canada, at least that I am aware.

I know it is common west of the divide in BC, Montana and Idaho, at higher elevations.

The large perennial is a member of the carrot family and easily mistaken at first for other white flowering members like angelica, or yampa.

One distinguishing trait, unlike other members of the Parsley family, is the dead plant material around the crown of the taproot. Another one, is the spicy, celery scent of the plant.

Various tribes used the dried root for sore throats and cold, either chewing on a small piece, or prepared as a tea.

For toothache, headache, stomachache, fever and heart issues, the root was chewed and the saliva slowly swallowed. The Cree traded with western Montana natives for the root, which they valued for heart problems.

Known as **QAWAQA'WS** to the Nez Perce, it was considered one of their most important medicines. The Blackfoot, Salish and other tribes describe it as Bear Medicine, in reference to observing bears utilize the root for their own healing.

In his book on Montana native uses of plants, Jeff Hart, recalls the use of the root for seizures as told by a Flathead woman.

"We get this root. We have to chew on it and just rub it on a person's body. We also rolled cigarettes with this root in it and let the person smoke it. That calms the seizure down."

The Flathead also believed that one shouldn't wash the root on site as that ensures a rainstorm. Considering the plant grows in moist, wet meadows and boggy slopes, the chances are it is raining as you are collecting the roots!

In fact, the strong-scented root was smoked, with tobacco, by the Secewepemc and Okanagan of British Columbia. They named it **XASXES**, meaning literally, "always good". It has been used traditionally in rituals and ceremonies for spiritual enlightenment and improved mental health.

The Crow used the root for the above uses, as well as use by singers to ensure vocal cords and throats did not give out during long ceremonies.

The root was shaved and added to boiling water as a steam treatment for sinus congestion and infection. A few shavings make a pleasant scented incense when added to some live coals.

MEDICINAL

CONSTITUENTS- roots and shoots- melatonin, serotonin, E-butylidenephthalide, Z-ligustilide, and ferulic acids. Work by Christina E. Turi & Susan J. Murch *Planta Medica* 2013 79:14 1370-9 detected more than 34000 compounds and 70 putative phthalide metabolites in plant.

It is often compared, in an unfavorable light, to its more famous cousin Osha (*L. porteri*). This is quite unfair, as the root, although smaller, is useful for many of the same diaphoretic and stimulating qualities.

The root, like Calamus, is rich in volatile oils that rapidly disperse in heat. Cold infusions or tinctures of the fresh root make the best medicine for treating various cold, flu and respiratory conditions, similar in some ways to Wild Ginger root.

It combines well with pleurisy root for inflamed lungs with thick yellow mucous, and you may add mallow root if too thick.

Canby's Lovage root is mildly anti-viral, and analgesic, and best chewed, in the traditional manner, for sore throats and bronchial problems.

It may be a mild uterine stimulant, so caution is advised during pregnancy, at least completely in first trimester. The root is said to attract bears and repels rattlesnakes.

The content of melatonin and serotonin in roots and shoots is suggestive of benefit in modulating brain activity.

RECIPES

Gather the roots in fall when foliage has died back. Slice and make a fresh root tincture at 1:3 and 60% alcohol. Dosage is from 1-5 ml as needed.

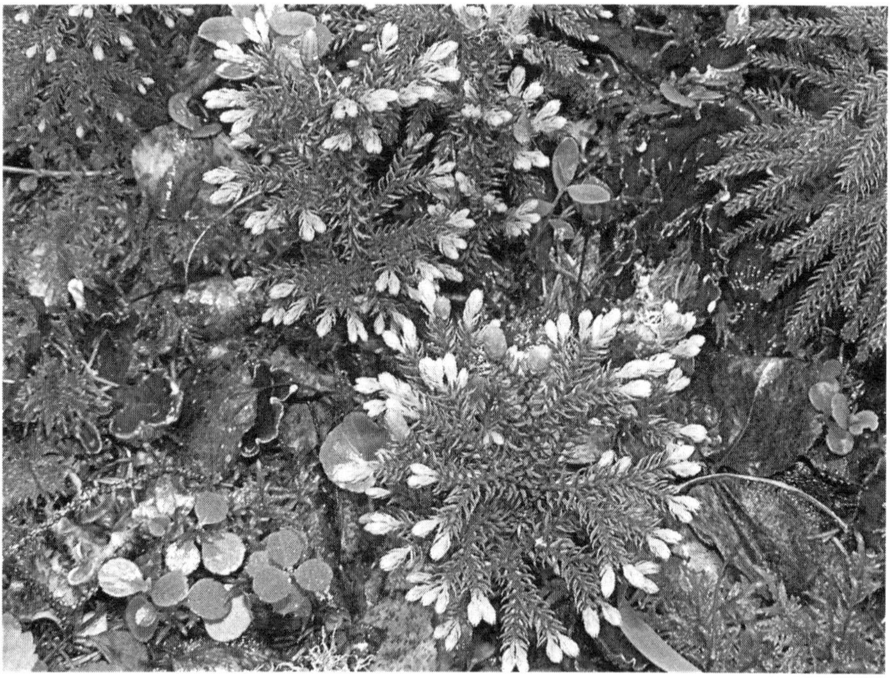

Ground Pine (*Lycopodium dendroideum*)

RUNNING CLUBMOSS
(*Lycopodium clavatum* L.)
GROUND CEDAR
(*L. complanatum* L.)
(*Diphasiastrum complanatum* L. [Holub])
(*Diphasium anceps*)
(*L. anceps*)
GROUND PINE
TREE CLUBMOSS
(*L. obscurum var. dendroideum* [Michx.] D.C. Eat.)
(*L. dendroideum* Michx.)
NORTHERN FIR CLUBMOSS
MOUNTAIN CLUBMOSS
(*L. selago* L.)
(*Huperzia selago* [L.] Bernh. ex Schrank & Mart.)

MOUNTAIN FIR CLUBMOSS
ALPINE FIR MOSS
(***H. haleakalae*** [Brackenridge] Holub.)
STIFF CLUBMOSS
BRISTLY CLUBMOSS
INTERRUPTED CLUBMOSS
(***L. annotinum*** L.)
(***L. dubium***)
NORTHERN BOG CLUBMOSS
(***L. inundatum*** L.)
(***Lycopodiella inundata***)

PARTS USED- spores, plant and root

The club-moss is on my person,
No harm or mishap can me befall;
No sprite shall slay me, no arrow shall wound me,
No fay nor dun water-nymph shall tear me.

ALEXANDER CARMICHAEL

Lycopodium is from the Greek **LYKOS**, meaning wolf, and **PODUS** for foot.

Club moss and its related genus and family are valuable medicinal plants that form fairy rings in fields and openings of the boreal forest. Inundatum means "apt to be flooded" and refers to a species that grows in bogs and moister regions of the boreal forest.

The Druids used the spores as a "cloth of gold" to protect them from black magic. Club moss is ruled over by the planets Saturn and Capricorn.

Druid nuns gathered the plant in the Loire Valley of France for their altars.

It had to be picked by a naked virgin with a newly woven cloth covering her hand and personifying the moon. She had to uproot the Selago with the tip of her little finger, after drawing a circle around it.

In some parts of Europe, club moss was believed to cause discord and argument when brought into groups. And yet, ironically, the Swedes use the stems for matting of Christmas wreaths.

While in Peru, I observed club moss species added to San Pedro cacti to enhance the hallucinogenic effect. Various species are known as Condor plant, in honor of the large bird. When added to San Pedro, the plant spirit appears to the Curandero as a Condor, which can astral travel. In this way, the healer can bring back the lost soul to a patient suffering from Susto, or fright. I observed this ceremony on more than one occasion while living in Peru. In Trujillo, the plant is known as *Trenza Shimbe*, and used to improve visionary sight. Another name is *Trencilla Verde*.

The spores are referred to as Flour of the Witches.

In Nepal, club moss is sacred to the Hindu god Vishnu, and used in ceremonies.

The Native people of Alberta used the yellow spore powder on wounds; inhaling them for severe nosebleeds. Steaming decoctions of white spruce needles and club moss were used for stiff joints in sweat lodges.

The Cree of northern Alberta call Running Clubmoss, **ASTASKAMKWA**.

Cree medicine used the spores as a metaphysical expression of a patient's health. Spores were placed on top of water; and if they radiated towards the sun, then the patient would survive. The waterproof property of spores was put to good use in separating fish eggs from the membranes in food preparation.

The Nitinaht of Vancouver Island considered it bad luck; and touching the plant would cause one to lose their way in the forest. The Tlingit word is **KUWAKAAN SIIGI** meaning "deer's belt".

The Gitksan call it **BELANA WATSX**, meaning belt of land otter. It was traditionally used to make wreaths for graves, as the otter is a powerful, spiritual animal, but one that can be dangerous and cause madness or death.

The spore powder or "witch's flour" is highly flammable, and was put to good use by early photographers and theatre prop artists; known as "vegetable cordite". It is source of the expression "flash in a pan". The powder was used in early stages of photocopy technology as well as forensic science.

A fun campfire trick is to quickly sprinkle some spores for a dramatic flash, something practiced by shaman from various cultures.

It has been previously used in hair powder, suppositories, surgical gloves and condoms. As many mature males are having their prostate health checked more frequently, it is best to use spore free gloves in rectal exams. These spores can cause allergic reaction in sensitive individuals; including hay fever, asthma and serious cell granuloma.

The Chinese use **SHEN JIN CAO** (*L. clavatum*) pollen as a dusting powder, to coat suppositories, and a dehumidifier to keep pills from sticking together. Decoctions of the plant are analgesic, and used for cramping, and arthritic complaints associated with painful joint movement. The herb is said to relax the tendons and circulate blood.

In the Himalayas, the whole plant and spores are taken internally for spasmodic retention of urine in infants, and externally for catarrhal cystitis.

In Africa, running clubmoss is mixed with *Selaginella rupestris* for headaches.

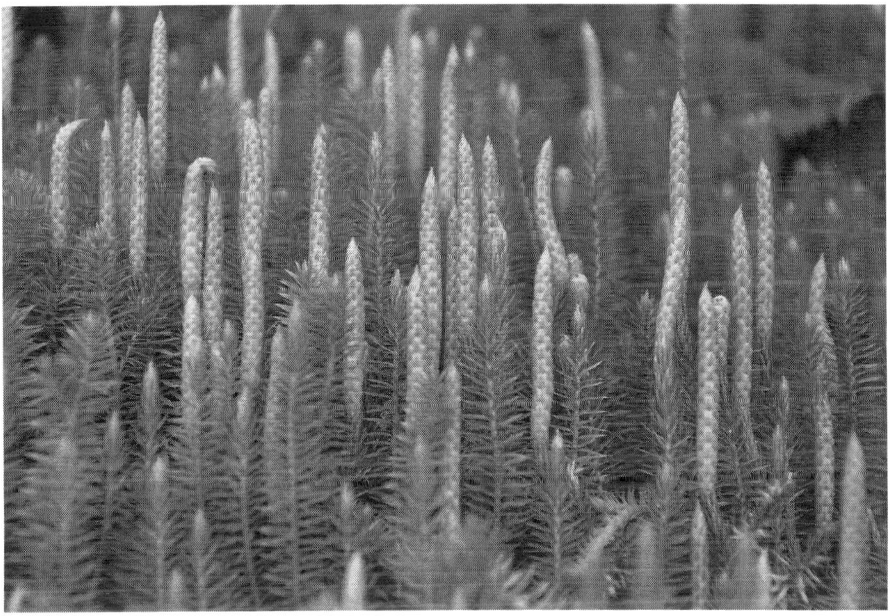

Stiff Clubmoss (*Lycopodium annotinum*)

Ground cedar decoctions were used by Blackfoot in the treatment of lung and venereal disease; very similar to its use by the Chinese. They used ground cedar spores for athlete's foot and fungal ulcers. The roots were a mordant or fixative for natural dyes like alum root.

Ground cedar (*L. complanatum*) was used traditionally by making a tea of the dried, powdered plant for increasing urine flow, starting delayed menstruation and relieving uterine spasms. The tea was used as an aphrodisiac. Further southeast, the Ojibwa used the dried leaves as a reviver; and the Iroquois used the herb as part of a combination decoction to induce pregnancy.

The herb contains stimulating effect, as opposed to the more narcotic *L. selago*.

The spores were boiled, and used as a hair wash for lice. The plant may live up to 850 years old.

Ground Pine (*L. obscurum*) spores were traditionally used, by the Chinese, as a desiccant for athlete's foot, and other fungal infections. The plant was decocted for spasmodic and analgesic conditions, like arthritis, back pain and nocturnal emissions.

Ground Pine was boiled and drunk as a purgative by the Montagnais in cases of biliousness. The Iroquois used cold decoctions for weak blood and root decoctions for the menopausal change of life.

The Flambeau used it along with Northern Bush Honeysuckle (*Diervilla lonicera*) as a diuretic; while the Chippewa used it with spruce twigs to steam rheumatic joints.

Fir club moss (*H. selago*) is chewed by Alaskan natives, as an intoxicant, to create a mild hypnotic and narcotic state. Northern and Mountain Clubmoss are similar, with the latter somewhat smaller, and found at higher elevation. Both have been called *L. selago* in the past; and were used by the Druids of Wales as an active cathartic and de-obstruent.

Women of the Scottish Highlands used the plant as an abortifacient. This is not surprising as women in Argentina use decoctions of the related *L. saururus,* known as Cola de quirquincho, for the same purpose.

William Emboden said that a tea from three stems will induce narcosis with small amounts both emetic and cathartic. In the Highlands of Scotland, it was taken in small doses to induce giddiness, and in larger amounts caused convulsion or miscarriage.

Fir Clubmoss was dried and ground as a dusting powder, or steeped and cooled for a softening lotion applied to skin.

Millspaugh wrote "it is also strongly counterirritant when applied to the skin, being used to keep blisters open, and to kill lice upon animals."

Huperzia species are without cones, and come in two forms often mistaken for two different species. One is short and thick, and another long and thinner, but neither creep on the ground.

Pliny mentions its use in treating uterine problems, knee problems, swollen thighs, water retention, and dropsy. One German name **BÄRLAPP** means uterine ointment.

It was listed in the *US Pharmacopoeia* as useful in absorbing fluids from injured tissue.

Smoke from dried club moss was used to treat eye disease in Highlands of Scotland. It was given internally, to treat glaucoma by Polish physicians in the 1940s.

The Inuit of Baffin Island and other northern islands used Stiff Club Moss for eye problems. The name **SIQPIIJAUTIT** means, "that which is used to remove siqpik," or discharge from the inner corner of the eye. The tops are very soft when ripe.

Inuit elders use it as an intoxicant that makes one dizzy and a light feeling in the head. It was boiled until the water turned black.

A recent article by Black et al, *Can J Botany* 2008 86 identified a broth containing Stiff Club Moss by the Inuit of Baffin Island, and *Oxyria digyna* for general health and hallucinogenic activity.

Mountain Sorrel (*O. digyna*) is known as **QUNGULIIT** by Inuit of Baffin Island.

Sporopollenin from *L. clavatum* has been found to be capable of acting as a solid support for peptide synthesis. In work by MacKenzie et al, *Int J Pept Protein Res* 1980 15:3 it was found to have numerous important practical advantages over synthetic resins.

Several authors believe that Clubmoss takes up astonishing amounts of aluminum from the soil. The ash is said to contain up to 30% of this metal.

This content of aluminum led to its replacement of the mordant alum (potassium aluminum sulphate) in fixing dyes. The colors are soft and less bright than alum but last longer.

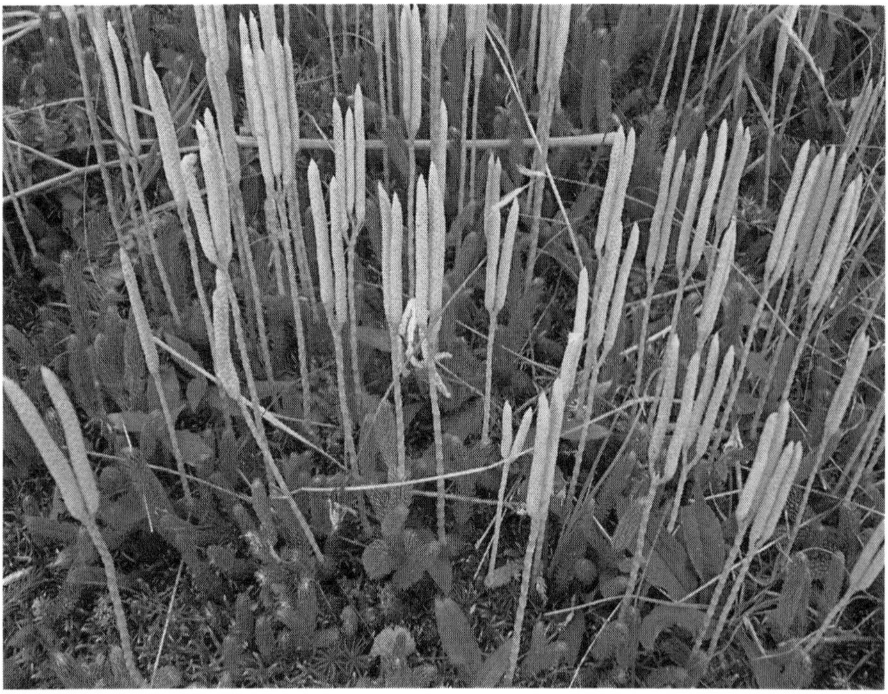

Clubmoss (Lycopodium clavatum)

MEDICINAL

CONSTITUENTS- *Lycopodium clavatum* spores- pollenin (45%), sporopollenin, decyl-isopropyl-acrylic acids, myristic acid, sporonine, lycopodine, radium, resins, 50% fatty acid, various decanoic acids, and flabelline.

The plant contains flavones, beta-sitosterol, clavatine, nicotine, lycopotine, fawcetine, fawcetimine, deactyl-fawcetine, clavatoxine, and apigenin-4'-O-beta-D-glucoside. It contains the alkaloids, fawcettimine, lycopodine, dihydro-lycopodine,

acetyldihydrolycopodine, alpha obscurine, clavolonine, lycodine and numerous triterpenoids including alpha onocerin, lyclaninol, lyclanitin, lyclavanol, lyclavinin, lyclavatol, lycocryptol, etc. Also contains vanillic, ferulic and azelaic acid, as well as 16-oxoseratenediol.
Ground cedar (*L. complanatum*) has similar spore composition.
The plant contains complanatine, lycopodine, alpha-obscurine, serra-tenediol, tohogenol, lyconadin A, complanadine D and nicotine.
Ground Pine (*L. obscurum*)- alpha & beta obscurine (diazaphenanthrene alkaloids).
Northern Fir Clubmoss (*L. selago*)- huperzine A (selagine) alkaloids including lycopodines, arifoline, serratidine, pseudo-selagine (isolycodoline) and lycodoline..
L. annotinum- alpha and beta obscurine, and various alkaloids including annofoline, annopodine, annotine, annotinine, isolycopodine, alpha and beta lofoline, lycodine, lycodoline, lycofawcine, lycofoline, lyconnotine, lycoposcrraminc M, anhydrolycodoline, gnidioidine, acrifoline, N oxide of annotine and lycopodine.
L. inundatum- dehydrolycopecurine, (-)-3-dehydro-trans-9-methyl-10-ethyl-lobelidiol, inundatine, isoinun-datine, lycopodine.

Club moss spore powder was previously used as a dusting powder for condoms, and a safe pharmaceutical aid to prevent pills sticking together.

It was a valuable body powder for the bedridden, known as Vegetable Sulphur, and dusted on bedsores, eczema, and herpes eruptions.

It excels for diaper rash, because it is not only soothing, but contains a waxy substance that is water repellent. If you coat your hand with spores and put it into water, your hand will remain completely dry!

Intertrigo, a dermatitis associated with moisture between skin folds, responds well to the soothing spore powder.

Fomentations of the plant, or pillows stuffed with the dry herb, relieve leg and foot cramps; and even headaches.

A tincture of the spores is recommended for extreme sensitivities of the skin. Slow, painful boils and swollen lymphatic nodes respond to the tincture.

Tinctures of the fresh plant, before it spores, sedate gastric disturbance, accompanied by blood filled urine. Painful urine retention by children and adults suffering from mucous filled, painful urination is helped.

Rheumatism and gout, with buildups of uric acid in the system and chronic kidney weakness with fevers are assisted.

Lycopine, an alkaloid of club moss, has been found to stimulate peristalsis, which encourages bowel movements. Lycopodine, however, produces uterine contractions and increases small intestinal peristalsis, so caution is advised.

Cirrhosis of the liver, accompanied by shortness of breath, responds to frequent infusions of the warm tea.

In China, the whole plant of *L. clavatum* is called **SHEN JIN CAO** meaning, "stretch the tendon herb", and is used to dispel wind and remove dampness. It relieves the rigidity of muscles, tendons and joints and dysmenorrhea. The herb is acrid, warm and dispersing.

For trauma related pain, combine with ground ivy.

When wine mix-fried, club moss is superior for dispelling wind, cold, dampness, and opening network blood vessels.

Studies by Orhan et al, in Turkey isolated alpha onocerin from *L. clavatum*, and found it to be a new acetyl-cholinesterase inhibitor, that may be useful in the treatment of Alzheimer's disease. *Planta Medica* 2003 69:3. Alpha onocerin has an IC50 of 5.2 mcg/M.

More recent work by same author, *J Ethnopharm* 109:1 found the alkaloid lycopodine, which comprises 85% of alkaloids, a powerful anti-inflammatory.

Clubmoss extracts exhibit acetyl-cholinesterase inhibition, at least in rat brain cortex, striatum and hippocampus. Konrath et al, *J Ethnopharm* 139:1.

In the Journal *Phytochemistry* 6:1 the same author found extracts active against *Staphylococcus aureus*, various fungi, and the *Herpes simplex* virus.

Work by Orhan et al, *Phytochem Rev* 2007 6 found activity against *S. aureus, Proteus mirabilis, Klebsiella pneumoniae, Acinetobacter baumannii* and *E. faecalis.* It possesses anti-viral effect against *herpes simplex* virus, similar to acyclovir, while an alkaloid fraction shows activity against para-influenza virus similar to oseltamivir. High antioxidant activity was noted as well.

Clubmoss extracts, *in vitro*, inhibit CYP3A4 liver enzymes, suggesting caution when combining with drugs. Tam et al, *Can J Physio Pharmacol* 2011 89:1.

Spore extracts show protective effects against various markers in mice, leading to liver tumors.

Reductions in glutathione reductase, hemoglobin, estradiol and testosterone, and increased blood glucose and cortisol were all normalized with administration. Pathakt et al, *Ind J Exp Biol* 2009 47:7.

Ground Cedar (*L. complanatum*) contains complanadine D, that enhances mRNA expression for NGF. The plant contains 61% lycopodine. Ether extracts show activity against anti-cholinesterase and butyrl-cholinesterase, as well as the *herpes simplex* virus. Orhan et al, *Nat Prod Res* 2009 23:6.

Fir club moss (*L. selago*) may be boiled and strained as an effective eyewash. The spores are used in China for uterine problems, swollen knees, thighs and ankles, and water retention.

Recent research indicates it may be effective treatment for herpes, myasthenia gravis and Alzheimer's disease- an exciting possibility! This is due to the discovery that *L. selago* contains selagine- a compound chemically identical to huperzine. Work by Dr. Alan Kozikowski at University of Pittsburgh has identified selagine as identical to huperzine.

Work by Feigenhauer et al, found Fir Club Moss water extracts to contain significant anti-cholinesterase activity. They found that the amount of huperzine A and B in *L. selago* was sufficient for relevant acetyl cholinesterase inhibition. *Journal Tox Clinical Toxicology* 2000 38:7. This followed from observing two patients who drank the herb tea by mistake, and experienced excess sweating, dizziness, and slurring of speech.

The related Chinese Clubmoss, **CHIEN TSENG TA**, or **SHUANG YI PING** (*L. serratum*) contains huperzine A, which is three times more potent than phytostigmine, as an acetyl-cholinesterase (AChE) inhibitor.

Other names for *Huperzia serrata* include, **QIAN CENG TA**, meaning "thousand layered pagoda", and **JIN BU HUAN**, "more valuable than gold". Indeed!

In clinical trials conducted by Cheng in 1986, it showed improvement in 98% of cases of myasthenia gravis; and improving memory in senile dementia. Content of huperzine A is highest in mid-fall and lowest in early spring.

It has shown in studies to decrease neuronal cell death caused by toxic levels of glutamate.

This makes huperzine A a potential medicine for reducing neuronal injury from strokes, epilepsy, and other disorders. For more information see *JAMA* Mar 12 1997.

Huperzine A shows NMDA receptor blocking, as well as anti-cholinesterase activity, and may be useful for prevention of epileptic seizures. Schneider et al, *Epilepsy Behav* 2009 July 16.

Huperzine A is a novel cognition enhancer, both inhibiting cholinesterase activity and modulating NMDA (N-methyl-D-aspartic acid) an excitatory amino acid transmitter. Both dementia and schizophrenia patients may benefit. Chiu et al, *J Compl Integr Med* 2007 4:1.

Huperzine B is reported in *Acta Pharm Sinica* 1999 20:2 to have anti-cholinesterase properties, is more selective than tacrine, and with less toxicity.

In one double-blind, randomized study, huperzine A was tested in 56 patients with senile dementia and 104 patients with senile and pre-senile simple memory disorders. The injectable form showed the most significant positive effects.

Another study of 50 Alzheimer's disease patients showed significant improvement in 58% of patients, in a multi-centre, randomized, double-blind, placebo-controlled study.

A placebo-controlled, double-blind study of 160 Alzheimer's patients found huperzine A significantly superior to placebo, tacrine and physostigmine, a cholinesterase inhibitor, with longer activity than the two drugs.

Huperizine A works on acetylcholine, only in the brain, giving it vast advantage over drugs such as cholinesterase inhibitors for Alzheimer's disease. It is non-toxic at up to 100 times human therapeutic dosage, and is an atropine antidote.

Huperizine A, when compared to tacrine, donepezil and rivastigmine, shows better penetration of the blood brain barrier, higher oral bioavailability and longer AChE inhibition.

John Heinerman used club moss herb in an energy and stamina formula. He added the plant because it contained some compounds that cross the blood brain barrier, and positively affect the limbic centre of the brain.

Ground Pine (*L. obscurum*) has been shown in clinical trials to contain anti-viral properties against the herpes simplex I implicated in cold sores.

Lycopodium spores were widely used in the 1920s as a dusting powder. If the spores found their way into surgical wounds they would cause granulation, even decades later, resembling cancerous or tuberculosis sores. The soothing, water resistant nature of the spores was put to use at one time in the treatment of intertrigo, a dermatitis caused by a build up of water between skin folds. The spores should not, however, be used externally on wounds.

The alkaloid fordine has been found in at least 14 species of *Huperzia*, and has similar action. All club moss in the boreal forest could be tested for this valuable compound.

In rat studies, fordine at 0.01-0.04 mg/kg IP speeds up conditioned avoidance responses, reverses impairment of conditioned avoidance response, and antagonizes hippocampal and cortical EEG changes induced by quinuclidinyl benilate.

Stiff club moss contains a number of alkaloids including annotine and lycodine that show activity noted above.

HOMEOPATHY

Lycopodium (*L. clavatum*) is one of our most valuable remedies. Patients that can benefit are prone to disorders of the digestive system often suffering from bloating and gas. They may sit down hungry, and yet a bite or two fills them up.

They may be awakened by hunger pains and headaches, if they don't eat when their body suggests. Meat, oysters, onions, cabbage, or milk may aggravate their symptoms.

One peculiar symptom is that one foot may be hot; but the other is cold. All symptoms are worse on the right side of the body and worse between 4 and 8 pm. A fan-like movement of the wings of the nostrils observed during breathing, suggests this remedy may be helpful in alleviating the above symptoms. There is a craving for sweets and warm drinks.

The male may be impotent, and the female have menses that are long and profuse. Vaginal dryness is irritated by sex.

Classically, the Lycopodium patient needs someone to be close, but not necessarily in the same room.

DOSE- For elimination try 2X or 3X, a few drops in water before meals. Use 4X for mood swings and desire for sweets, related to both physiological and psychological issues.

Higher potency is for mental and emotional symptoms. Try 30X for babies that sleep all day and cry all night. The mother tincture is prepared from the spores, gathered towards the end of summer. The powder is pale yellow, and both odorless and tasteless.

The first three attenuations are made by mixing one grain of powder to one hundred grains of milk sugar, for 1X.

For higher potencies, the 1X powder can be diluted in alcohol. Work by Pathak et al, *Forsch Komple* 14:3 found Lycopodium 200, as alcohol extraction, possesses liver cancer fighting potential.

MATERIA POETICA

You are bossy, so I see
Boaster, braggart, class bully
I didn't like your puffed up shirt
Treating me like I was dirt
Then I saw you acquiesce
Act so meek and kiss her feet
I wondered what was going on
First you've got an awful bark
Then you snivel in the dark
Outside big and inside small
What a split that fooled us all
Afraid of trying something new
Afraid someone is watching you
Afraid your body's on the blink
Sudden weeping when you're thanked
Your tummy rumbles full of air
Like your ego making noise
Thirsty, hungry, food's your fare
Eating sweets, life's simple joys
On your right the problem starts
Then to the left and with a fart
Lycopodium don't be a bore
Early mornings and at 4
Take your remedy today
Before your hair starts turning gray!

SYLVIA CHATROUX

SPORE OIL

The spores of *L. clavatum* contain about 50% fat. This fat is interesting, in that its fatty acids contain only a small proportion of saturated acids, and more than 90% of the liquid acids are monoethenoic acids. About 30% of the total fatty acids consist of 9-hexadecenoic acid, according to work by Reibsomer and Johnson.

Lycopodium oil has been prepared by extracting the spores with chloroform with a saponification value of 195, and iodine value of 91.8. The oil is a bright yellowish-green. It does not solidify, even at -15° Celsius.

The oil, according to Rathje, contains 81% lycopodic acid, 3.2% dihydroxystearic acid, and small amounts of stearic, myristic and palmitic acid.

Various *Lycopodium* species contain lipids in both the runners and spikelets. Here is a brief synopsis:

Total lipids- *D. complanatum* runners, 39 mg/g, with spikelets, 87; *H. selago*, 89-202 mg/g; *L. annotinum* 72-202.

In the neutral lipids, *H. selago* stands out with 29.4 % diacylglycerol (DAG), but all contain mono- di and tri-cylyglycerols, as well as free sterols, sterol esters, alcohols, and waxes.

Interestingly, *D. complantum* is highest in phospholipids, including phosphatidyl choline and phosphatidyl ethanol-amine. *Chemistry of Natural Compounds* 2002 38:5.

LICHEN ESSENCES

Stiff Clubmoss essence teaches us to exist in spite of adversity, and gives courage in times of set backs or resignation. **MARIANA**

Clubmoss spore essence is for those people who have great fear of being alone. They are intellectually keen, but physically slow and underdeveloped. In social circles, they worry what other may think of them. They can never be satisfied, and can be stubborn, ungrateful and dictatorial.

They try to hide their insecurity by bluff and bravado; being domineering to those younger, weaker or less intelligent. They may have fear of the dark, crowds, speaking in public, and even death.

PRAIRIE DEVA

PERSONALITY TRAITS

Clubmoss people are of keen intellect, with weak muscular power. They have a dry temperament with dark complexions.

The dryness results from excessive mental activity; while decreased glandular and lymphatic activity affects the liver and adrenal function.

Intellectually keen children, with high nervous tension and weak physicality, they may feel inferior and insecure. They may compensate for their weakness by exaggerating their strengths.

Carried to extreme, this is the "bookworm", or brooding introvert. And while this philosophical life may lead to highly, evolved spiritual values; it may also create neurotic, and self-centered goals. The result may be easily offended, intolerant, over bearing and domineering personalities. They are usually smokers.

Often, sexual capacity is reduced, with incomplete erection and difficult ejaculation.

Indeed, the characteristics of the plant compare favorably with those who can use it.

Clubmoss is of dry and thin growth, creeping shyly along the ground. The spores repel water (emotion), are extremely hard; and burn with a very bright flash.

The spores germinate after 6-7 years, and the plant reaches maturity at 12-15 years.

The living dynamics of the herb are expressed as dryness, slowness, hardness with hidden, fiery qualities, and yet a great hesitance to grow and reproduce.

PRAIRIE DEVA

[Clubmoss types] are charming, intellectual, and ambitious, and struggle with sexuality and commitment. They are well known as dictators in their work or at home but at the other end of the scale can be very timid in all situations. They commonly display both traits in differing situations. Their love of power makes them poor team players, as they prefer to be at the top.

Being essentially ambitious academics rather than practical types, they are found in professions rather than business, often at the top of a partnership or committee. They think they are equal players, but to everyone else they act like the boss. They give the idea of a petty tyrant rather than a warlord. They exaggerate and puff up their intellectual and other abilities to make themselves look better and more capable than they are.

They can be tyrannical children and even before they speak they boss the parents around. When older they can take the lead role and tell the others what they are doing wrong.

Or they can be introverted type, cautious and fearful of normal playground behavior, and can become absorbed in safe, intellectual activities such as reading and computers.

According to their type they can be either the bullied or the bully.

Commitment is a major issue for *Lycopodium*, because they find that their passion is short lived (dry emotions); so they can thrive on affairs but not easily in marriage. The man may decide not to marry; or once the children have arrived and he is no longer top of the list in his wife's affections, he may run off with his secretary, who restores him to top place and massages his ego projections (confident at work, uncertain at home). One problem that can plague him is his anticipatory anxieties and cowardice underneath, leading to failing erections.

PETER CHAPPELL

The central theme of the *Lycopodium* remedy pattern is a lack of confidence. People in this pattern are sensitive to criticism. These stresses and anxieties can make them irritable. They tend to complain when they feel overburdened with responsibilities and sometimes they try to shirk them. They feel trapped if they have all the financial responsibility for their dependents, and they can be grudging with money as well as with time spent with their families.

Lycopodium helps you feel more confident and secure in your own power. Your experience of power was that it was imposed from the outside, which made you believe that the only way to be strong was to strive for power over others. **LORIUS**

MYTHS AND LEGENDS

It was gathered with great care, no iron instrument was allowed to touch it, even bare hands were unworthy of this honor. A special covering, or "sagus" was used with the right hand. This covering had to be consecrated and secretly received from a holy personage with the left hand. It could be collected only by a white clad druid, with bare feet, that had been washed in clear water.

Before he collected this plant, he had to make an offering of bread and wine; after this, the plant was carried away from the place in which it grew in a new, clean cloth.

In the "Kadir Taliesin", selago is referred to as "the gift of god", and in modern Welsh as the "gras duw", or the "grace of god". **SCHOPF**

Once when were children we stayed up late. The oldest person in our group boiled some plants over a fire at night. He made this brew. He gave us some and we drank it. After that I lay down and couldn't get up for quite a while. I was mentally aware of my surroundings but whenever I moved, I became really dizzy. When I tried to get up, I would fall forward. It think that we were drunk. Even after quite some time passed, I could not get up.

Those plants (*L. annotinum*) are intoxicating substances.

MALAIJA (OOTOOVA ET AL)

RECIPES

INFUSIONS- Pour one litre of boiling water over one tbsp of herb. Take small sips, on empty stomach, before meals. One to two cups daily.

TINCTURE- One teaspoon every three to four hours in water. The mother tincture for homeopathy is made from the powder of spores gathered at summer's end at a 2:1 with 95% alcohol.

The spores are considerable work to collect. The spikes are best picked in late summer and placed in a glass jar. They will mature in there and the occasional shake will have them fall to the bottom. Trying to shake a little at a time into a paper bag has never worked well for me, especially when it may be cold and snowing at the same time as sporulation in northern Alberta.

HUPERZINE A- 100-150 mcg twice daily or 2 microgram per kilo of patient weight.

CAUTION- Do not use during pregnancy, or with hypertension, liver or kidney disease, epilepsy, asthma, IBS or irregular heart.

It may increase the effects of acetyl-cholinesterase inhibitors such as tacrine, and anti-cholinergic drugs such as bethanechol.

PILLOW- Fill a small bag with the newly dried club moss. Apply as needed.

DECOCTION- Use the entire plant including root. For dyes, combine root with the natural plant and boil together.

WILD DAFFODIL
(*Narcissus pseudo-narcissus* L.)
CHINESE SACRED LILY
TAZETTA DAFFODIL
(*N. tazetta* L.)
JONQUIL
(*N. jonquilla* L.)
NARCISSUS
(*N. poeticus* L.)
PARTS USED- bulb, flower

Who comes into this country and has come where golden crocus and narcissus bloom, where the great Mother, mourning for her daughter and beauty drunken by the water. **W.B. YEATS**

But I, beloved Narcissus, am only curious
About my own essence;
For me, everything else is only a mystery
Everything else is only absence. **PAUL VALERY**

Daffodils yellow, daffodils gay
To put upon the table on Easter day.
I wandered lonely as a cloud that floats on high o'er vales and hills,
When all at once I saw a crowd, a host, of golden daffodils.
WM WORDSWORTH

The Narcissus wondrously glittering, a noble sight for all, whether immortal gods or mortal men; from whose root a hundred heads spring forth, and at the fragrant odor thereof all the broad heaven above and all the earth laughed, and the salt wave of the sea. **HOMER**

To love oneself is the beginning of a life-long romance.
OSCAR WILDE

Narcissus is either from the Greek **NARKAO**, meaning to benumb, or **NARKISSOS**, a beautiful boy in myths. Narcotic, and narcolepsy are from the same root.

In Greek mythology, Narcissus was a beautiful youth loved by the goddess Echo. The flower scent was used by Pluto to lure Proserpine into hell and by ancient Greeks to subdue the dark spirits. Socrates called it the "Chaplet of the infernal Gods", due to its narcotic effects.

Daffodil is a corruption of **AFFODYL** from the Greek **ASPHODELOS**, the flower they believed bloomed in the afterlife.

The Asphodel, mentioned in ancient poetry, turned into the Middle Dutch, **DE AFFODIL** and into English in that manner.

Other authors suggest the name is a corruption of Dis's Lily, as it is the flower supposed to have dropped from the chariot of that God, in his flight with Proserpine. This is a stretch, even for me!

Both Pliny and Theophilus mention Asphodels that grow beside the river Acheron in the underworld, bringing joy to the land of the dead.

Jonquillo is the Spanish diminutive of Junco, associated with the rush-like stems. Junkwill is the original pronunciation but in the 19th century it became John Quill, a better sounding name.

Daffodil symbolizes chivalry, and the birth date of February 17th. Yellow Daffodil (*N. pseudonarcissus*) is one of the national emblems of Wales.

White daffodil (*N. tazetta*) has been found in funeral wreaths on Egyptian mummies from circa 1570 BC. It later migrated east to Japan, India and China, where it is called the "Good Luck Flower", or "New Year Lily".

The Roman poet, Ovid, wrote out a recipe for "every woman who covers her face with this will make it more brilliant than a mirror." See below.

The daffodil is a favourite of prairie gardens and lawns. Its bright yellow face reminds us of spring, but few of us think of its medicinal use.

The Cree call the introduced plant **MEYOSKAMIN WAPIKWAN**.

Historically, the bulbs were boiled and used as an emetic. Poultices were made from the bulbs and applied to hard swellings, wounds, burns, sprains and joint pain, to numb the area and entire nervous system.

Hippocrates, the father of medicine, knew about the anti-cancer activity of Daffodil nearly 2400 years ago. Dioscorides and Soranus of Ephesus (AD 98-138) wrote of its early use. Pliny the Elder wrote of the topical use of extracts for cancer as well. Kornienko et al, *Chem Rev* 2008 108.

Early physicians used both the bulbs and flowers as anti-spasmodic for treating epilepsy and hysteria. They believed the bulb contained an alkaloid similar to atropine in action.

Back in 1627, the herbalist Parkinson had identified 80 different varieties of narcissus. These began to disappear and by the late 1800s there were few varieties.

Peter Barr began to travel the world collecting varieties and sending them back to Great Britain. At the age of 72, he went on a five-year tour of the world and became known as the Daffodil King.

In Victorian times, daffodil signified regard, and narcissus, conceit, vanity and egotism. In China, the former signifies purity and soul.

Other European physicians used it for intermittent fever, diarrhea, dysentery, worms, and severe catarrh.

In Elizabethan times, dried daffodil bulb and barley powder was applied to assorted skin eruptions and discolorations. The bulbs were also simmered in oil, and the resultant mixture applied to rough skinned heels.

The flowers have also been dried and powdered and used traditionally as emetics. In France, the flowers were used traditionally as an antispasmodic.

In Arabia, the flower oil was applied to cure baldness and as an aphrodisiac. In Arab poetry, the stalk represents a man standing or a devoted servant.

The bulb has been infused, or made into syrups that help pulmonary congestion, and bronchitis.

When introduced to China, narcissus was known as **SHIU XIAN**, the immortal from the water.

None of this is recommended, but noted for historical value. The bulbs of Wild Daffodil are poisonous. Do not consume. It has been noted that European badgers bring daffodil leaves and other fresh greens as bedding material to their den near birthing time.

Work by Barkham in the *Journal of Ecology* 1980 68 estimates a life span for wild daffodil is 120-180 years.

Daffodils are the floral emblem of the Canadian Cancer Society that, ironically, spends zero dollars on herbal and other plant-based medical research.

The use of daffodil as a floral emblem of Wales is recent, and a reaction to the traditional leek. An ancient Welsh belief is that whomever finds the first daffodil of spring will gain gold in a short time.

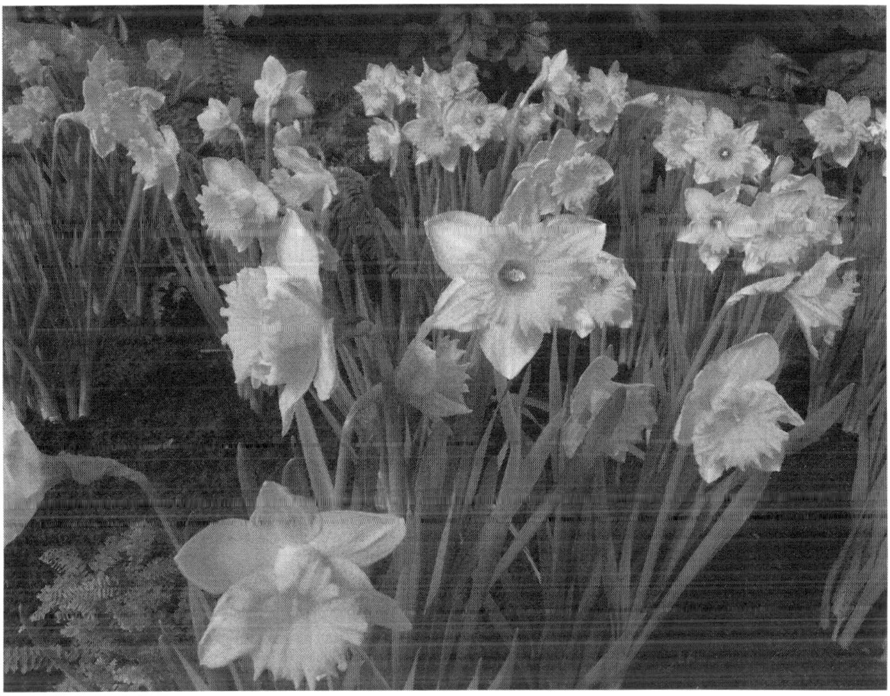

Daffodils

MEDICINAL

CONSTITUENTS- flowers- narcissine (lycorine)
leaf- amaryllidacene alkaloids including haemanthamin, galanthine, galanthamine, pluviin, masonine, homo-lycorin; as well as chelidonic acid.
bulbs- lycorine (narcissine), narcidine, galanthamine (3.9-78.7 mg/100 grams dry wt), masonine, irahine, homolycorin, oduline, pseudolycorine, suisemine, tazettine, narzettine, nartazine, haemanthanmine, fiancine, hippeastrine, galanthine, panceratine, narcissidine and a lectin known as agglutinin (NPA), narcissin, and calcium oxalate.
In resting bulbs, daffodil exhibits pilocarpine activity, while in flowering bulbs, atropine-like activity is present. Lycorine content is 0.2% in resting bulbs and 0.1% in flowering bulbs.
N. poeticus- bulb- galanthamine, lycorine, pancracine.
N. tazetta- lycorine, lycorenine, homolycorine, lycoramine, pseudo-lycorine, lycoranolidine, demethyl-homolicorine, lycoranoline, tazettine ($C_{18}H_{21}NO_5$), isotazettine, pluviine.
Narcissine was first isolated in 1578.

Daffodil leaves and flowers are used for irritations of the mucous membranes. These include bronchial catarrh, colds, asthma and even whooping cough.

Suzuki et al, *Proc Soc Expl Biol Medicine* 1974 145 looked at the therapeutic activity of Daffodil alkaloids on Rausher leukemia. The anti-viral activity and its use as part of drug combinations is of some interest. This was follow-up to work by a colleague in issue 1972 140.

Narcissine, a crystalline alkaloid is now called lycorine, after being isolated from the plant *Lycoris radiata*. Lycorine is an isoquinolone (phenathridine derivative) that acts as an emetic. It was first isolated in 1578, and in 1910 purified from bulbs yielding 0.1%. It possesses choline-mimetic effects.

Galanthamine is a cholinesterase inhibitor that exhibits analgesic activity.

In one study, extracts containing masonin and lomolycorin were found to induce delayed hypersensitivity in lab animals. NPA, the lectin, binds to alpha2-macroglobulin and to glycoprotein 120 of the HIV, *in vitro*.

It is inhibitory of HIV-1 and HIV-2, and cytomegalovirus infections.

This led scientists to believe the plant had potential for biochemical research, and new directions for AIDS research. Weiler et al, *J Gen Virol* 1990 71:1.

Various isoquinolone alkaloids including narcislasine, lycoricidine, lycorine, and isonarciclasine exhibit consistent activity against flaviviruses and bunyaviruses. Lycorine inhibits poliomyelitis virus at 1.0 mcg/ml.

This initial work by Balzarini et al, was reported in *Antimicrobial Agents and Chemotherapy* 1991 35.

Lycorine has been found to induce apoptosis in human leukemia (Jurkat) cell lines. McNulty et al, *Phytochem* 70:7.

Lycorine shows cytotoxic activity against *Trichomonas vaginalis*, suggesting a useful douche for this troublesome infection. Giordan et al, *Phytochem* 2011 72:7 645-50.

NPA inhibits rabies virus attachment to susceptible cells as well as rubella virus replication *in vitro*, in studies conducted by Balzarini et al, 1991.

NPA is used in biochemical research for its ability to bind with gluco-conjugates occurring on viruses such those above, as well as simian immunodeficiency virus.

It has been used to develop novel enzyme immunoassays for quantitation of envelope glycoprotein 120 on HIV.

Irehine, from narcissus bulbs, and boxwood, is used as a precursor to synthesize steroids.

Galanthamine is a tertiary amine alkaloid present in both common daffodils as well as snowdrops. It inhibits, reversibly, the enzyme acetyl-cholinesterase which breaks down acetylcholine, and may stimulate the brain's receptors to release more. Galanthamine has been reported effective in treating the mood disorder mania. It rapidly crosses the blood brain barrier.

Galanthamine increases frequency of opening nicotinic receptor channels, and potentiates agonist-activated receptors. It binds to an allosteric site on the alpha subunits of nicotinic acetylcholine receptors.

Galanthamine possesses analgesic properties possibly due to similarity in structure to codeine.

Daffodil lectins have been found to inhibit hepatoma, choriocarcinoma, melanoma and osteosarcoma cancer cell lines. Wang et al, *Int J Biochem Cell Biol* 2000 32:3.

More information on this alkaloid, undergoing clinical trials for treating Alzheimer's disease, can be found under Snowdrops, below. Reminyl is one such drug.

Two Daffodil cultivars show significant galanthamine content; Ice Follies at 76 mg and Mount Hood at 59 mg per 100 grams of dry weight. Initial work was from the variety King Alfred. The variety Carlton is grown under stressed conditions for commercial production. Lycorine was initially produced from the variety Twink.

Various Narcissus species contain the sparingly water-soluble anti-cancer isocarbostyril. Work by Pettit et al, *J Natural Products* 2003 66:1 found an efficient procedure to convert this into narcistatin, which shows activity against a range of human cancer cell lines.

Narciclasine is cytotoxic and its derivative, 7-deoxy-trans-dihydro-narciclasine strongly inhibits various cancer cell lines. Narciclasine, and indeed the whole daffodil, placed into a vase of water with other flowers will help them last longer.

Narcissin is also found in canola, lily species, puncture vine, sea buckthorn and European larch.

Trans-dihydronarciclasone is a readily available molecule with potent and selective anti-cancer activity based on Canadian work published in *Journal Nat Products* 2010 November 24.

The Tazetta Daffodil bulb (*N. tazetta*) is used in treating hypertension.

In Traditional Chinese Medicine, the bulb is known as **SHUI HSIEN KEN**. The bulb has a bitter, pungent flavor and acts on both the heart and lung meridians.

It has been used traditionally for dispelling heat, expelling wind and draining pus. It is also mashed and applied to insect bites, as well as more serious carbuncles, furuncles, boils, abscesses and mastitis.

The leaves contain a mannose binding lectin that exhibits hemagluttinating activity in studies with rabbit erythrocytes.

This same lectin shows activity against respiratory syncytial virus and various strains of influenza A (H1N1, H3N2, H5N1) and B viruses. Ooi et al, *J Bio Sci* 2010 35:1.

Crude plant extracts exhibit uterine stimulating and contracting effect.

Various alkaloids exhibit inhibitory effect on myoma tumors and Ehrlich ascites cancer.

Another extract treats viral-induced lymphocytic choriomeningitis. Isotazettine shows significant anti-tumour activity against the Rauster leukemia virus.

Tazettine has a melting point of 210° F.

Recent work by Evidente et al, *Phytochem Rev* 2009 8 looked at a variety of related alkaloids and their anti-cancer potential.

HOMEOPATHY

Narcissus (Daffodil) bulbs contain an alkaloid that varies whether the bulb is processed before or after flowering.

When processes before, it produces dryness of mouth, checks cutaneous secretions, dilates the pupil of the eye, quickens the pulse, and slows and weakens the heart contractions.

On the other hand, the alkaloid from the bulb after flowering, produces copious salivation, increases cutaneous secretion, contracts the pupil of the eye, produces slight relaxation of the pulse, and slight faintness and nausea.

Narcissus is a remedy for cough and bronchitis, with continuous coughing, nasal drainage and frontal headaches. It can be used in good service in the convulsive stage of whooping cough.

It relieves erythema of a papular, vesicular and pustular type, especially if aggravated by wet weather.

It should be thought of in gastro-enteritis with griping and cutting bowel pain.

DOSE- First attenuation.

A case of toxicology from eating a salad of narcissus (*N. poeticus*) and onion bulbs in 1844 resulted in observation of the following symptoms, reported in Allen.

Stupefaction, nausea, griping and burning pain in stomach, with gastroenteritis in second day after profuse vomiting. Small and trembling pulse, trembling of limbs, fainting, cold sweat and cold extremities.

ESSENTIAL OIL

Although there is no Daffodil or Narcissus essential oil, an absolute is produced in Europe from *Narcissus poeticus*. This is a late spring whitish flower hardy to zone 3-4.

The absolute is extremely expensive, and used for fine perfume blending. Narcissus oil was used in early Arabic perfumes, the scent in large amounts almost intoxicating.

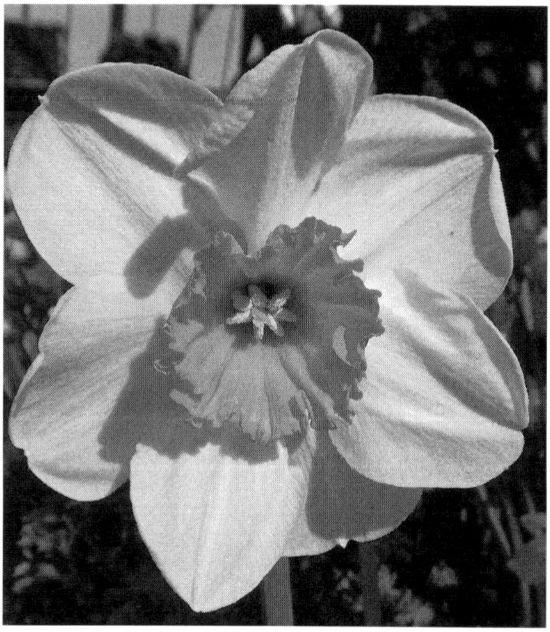

Daffodil

The Sufi say, "smell a narcissus, even if only once a day or once a week or once a month or once a year or once a lifetime. For verily in the heart of man there is the seed of insanity, leprosy and leukoderma. And the scent of narcissus drives them away".

Narcissus is used in aromatherapy for creating calm and deep relaxation that allows one delve deeply into the psyche, and confront your deepest fears.

The absolute is a dark green-orange colour, or occasionally dark olive, and somewhat grainy if not all the waxes are removed in final alcohol washing.

It blends well with clove bud, carnation, jasmine, neroli, ylang, rose, and mimosa, but is a difficult oil to bring out the best. It is both green, and earthy, and floral sweet all at the same time.

Rarely, an enfleurage is offered, but the price can easily be in the ten to twelve thousand dollar range per kilo, when available.

Chinese Sacred Lily (*N. tazetta*) is cultivated in the south of France for its oil, produced by either enfleurage or most likely, volatile solvents.

An analysis of an essential oil from the flower showed 61% trans ocimene.

The absolutes are used in about 11% of the finest modern perfumes, the notes faintly noticeable in Fatale and Samsara.

You may find it at the best Aromatherapy shops, but do not confuse it with the cheap fragrance oils that go by the same name. The price will advise you to authenticity.

FLOWER ESSENCES

Narcissus (*N. pseudo-narcissus*) flower essence is for the identification and resolution of conflicts by going to the centre of the problem or fear. From there, the issues can be faced by determining what is essential and nurturing to the Self.

It affects the root chakra, by helping us feel grounded. Physically, it promotes digestion, and helps with digestive disorders including excessive stomach acid, ulcer, gas and belching. **PACIFIC**

Jonquil (*N. poeticus*) flower essence is for the individual that believes " it will never be the same again", and is especially useful for children in fear, or uncertainty.

The essence helps give assurance that all will be well, with emotional and mental stability. **NEW ZEALAND**

Daffodil (*N. ajax*) flower essence extends the conscious mind's activity through the mental body, which it helps to organize, to certain levels of the higher self. This is desirable because the high self is actually a fine attunement of all the subtle bodies, and it is never out of harmony.

Daffodil vitalizes the body. This does not mean physically rejuvenating the body; it is more a vitality that manifests from a clarity of thought.

It is excellent for treating manic depression, psycho-spiritual imbalances, extreme frustration, low intellectual capacities, and constant self- condemnation.

The ability to grow plants under difficult conditions and all types of crop rotation will be enhanced with this essence.

GURUDAS

SPIRITUAL PROPERTIES

Narcissus is the slayer of internal dragons, the little voices of fear which surface when life experiences seem to be a cycle of endless challenges. It helps us to digest experiences and use them for further growth. It calms that feeling of "butterflies in the Stomach".

In Chinese medicine, the earth element requires support through nourishment. In the healthy stomach channel the energy flows downwards from heaven to earth.

When this flow is disrupted due to undigested ideas or emotions, there is a tendency for the energy flow to reverse and disturb the mind. This imbalance manifests as a preoccupation with details and obsessive thinking. **PETTITT**

The stem of the Daffodil is hollow like a wand. A wand is a tool that the Magician uses to create what he desires in life. It is a clear channel for the free-flowing energy between the flower's yellow crown that symbolizes Heaven and the round bulb that symbolizes Earth...We are the wands creating our own realities. The more discriminating we are in choosing the words we speak or the ideas we fill our minds with, the more likely we are to create what we desire. **RUDGINSKY**

Narcissus represents that beauty is not sufficient in itself, but wants to become divine as well. **THE MOTHER**

Narcissus has a spiritual quality and a flair for dissolving different boundaries, breaking through mental and spiritual blockages. This personality can be very persuasive, seductive and broad-minded. It despises pettiness, while loving freedom, joy, laughter and fun. It clears away low self-esteem. **VIVIAN LUNNY**

PERSONALITY TRAITS

Seven creamy white petals open to show a golden orange fluted cup in the centre. In traditional Tarot cards, the suit of Cups represent feelings and emotions. Narcissus looks as if it is smiling at the world, gracefully digesting experience. Its keynote, however, is its sweet perfume which can permeate a holy house, bringing calmness and peace of mind. **PETTITT**

Narcissus personalities have freedom of mind and consciousness and there are no ties that can bind them down or hold them back.

Narcissus personalities are what one might call "relaxed passionates". In love they'll be both tender and passionate and love both physically and spiritually…it seems that the Narcissus personality needs acclaim, kudos, and even exaltation, when in negative mode. This is when their egos become very fragile and Narcissus becomes self-effacing, self-limiting, and doubting of the intuition they previously trusted.

VALERIE WORWOOD

MYTHS AND LEGENDS

Narcissus was so handsome that he spurned the love of women and men. But one day beside a forest pool, the lad found his true love, himself, while gazing into the water.

He kept reaching to grasp his own reflection in the water, but each time he touched the surface, his image disappeared He could not bring himself to leave the bank of the pool and so he stayed there, forgetting to eat, entranced by his own beauty. When he eventually expired, the gods turned him into a golden flower. **CASSELMAN**

There was a Christianized version of Narcissus, said to have been a bishop of Jerusalem in the 2nd century A.D. He was credited with the usual long life (116 years) that early Christians claimed their religion could bring about. At the time of St. Narcissus, however, the Jerusalem temple was dedicated to Venus and her dying god Adonis, for whom Narcissus was an alternate name.

Jerusalem had no bishops. It has been suggested that the six petaled flowerets of narcissi stood for the six lobed symbol of Venus and the sacred hexagram that used to imply sexual union between Goddess and God. **WALKER**

Legend tells of a poor old widow who was saving her last half bowl of rice for her feckless son, when a hungry beggar appeared requesting food. Out of pity she gave him the rice; as he finished it he spat out a few grains and vanished. In the morning the old woman found that the rice grains had been transformed into a narcissus in full bloom, and promptly found fame and fortune by selling the plants. Since then, *N. tazetta* has represented prosperity and benevolence. **GRIMSHAW**

Demeter's daughter was gathering flowers over a soft meadow, roses and crocuses and beautiful violets, irises also and hyacinths and the narcissus which Earth made to grow at the will of Zeus and to please the Host of Many, to be a snare for the bloom-like girl—a marvelous, radiant flower. It was a thing of awe whether for deathless gods or mortal men to see; from its root grew a hundred blossoms and it smelled most sweetly, so that all wide heaven above and the whole earth and the sea's salt swell laughed for joy." **HOMER**

RECIPES

POWDER- 10-30 grains of powdered flowers decocted in 200 ml of water as an emetic. Let stand for 20 minutes.

EXTRACT- 2-3 grains as needed as emetic.

TINCTURE- 1 10 drops in water. The tincture is prepared from the fresh bulb in 98% alcohol.

GALANTHAMINE- Single doses of 10 mg are tolerated by humans without side effect. Maximum levels are present two hours after ingestion, with a half life of 5.3 hours, with bioavailability of 65-100%.

OVID'S POWDER- Finely powder equal parts of dried daffodil bulbs, barley and lentils, and make a paste by adding honey and water.

CAUTION- By no means are daffodil bulbs edible. Poisonings, including one death have been reported. Two children became ill after eating the leaves.

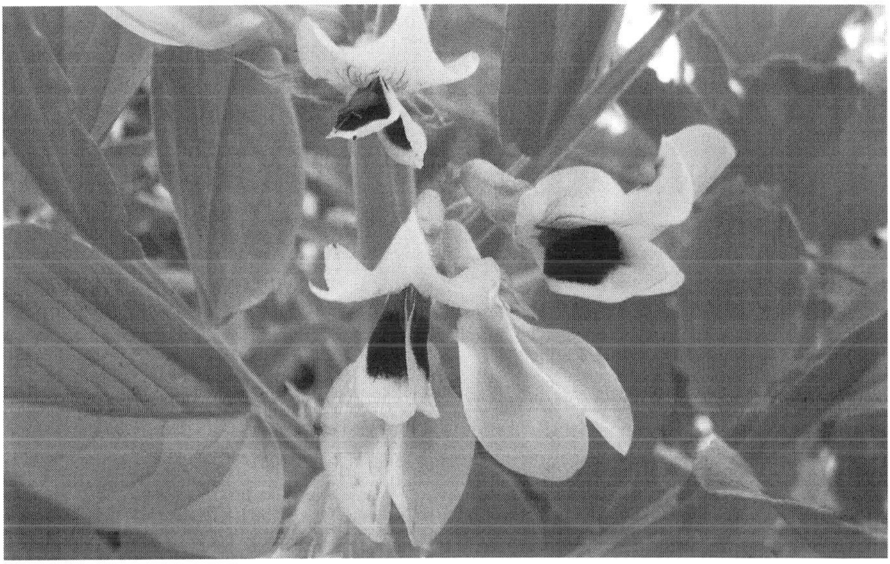

Faba Bean flowers

FAVA BEAN
FABA BEAN
WINDSOR BEAN
HORSEBEAN
BROADBEAN
MOJO BEAN
(***Vicia faba*** L.)
TICKBEAN
(***V. faba*** L.)
CRIMSON FLOWERING FAVA
(***V. faba*** L.)
ALPINE MILK VETCH
WILD VETCH
(***V. americana*** Muhl ex Willd)
(***V. sparsifolia*** Ten.)
TUFTED VETCH
(***V. cracca*** L.)
WOOLLY VETCH
HAIRY VETCH
(***V. villosa*** Roth)
(***V. dasycarpa*** Ten.)
PARTS USED- seed, flower

Beans are the substance which contains...that animated matter of which our souls are particles. **DIOSGENES**

First he ate some lettuce and some broad beans, then some radishes, and then, feeling rather sick, he went to look for some parsley.
BEATRIX POTTER, THE TALE OF PETER RABBIT

There was once a nest in a hollow,
Down in the mosses and knot grass pressed.
Soft and warm, and full to the brim,
Vetches hung over it purple and dim,
With buttercup buds to follow. **ANON**

Vicia is from thc Latin **VINCIO**, to bind. Vctch is thought to be corruption derived from the same root. Villosa means soft hairs, referring to the covered pods. Fava is an English corruption of Latin faba, meaning bean.

Faba beans were cultivated for over 6,000 years before *Phaseolus* beans reached the Old World. They reached China several thousand years later, and then moved to Japan and India.

The Israelites were familiar with faba and called them **POL** (Samuel II 17:18); which the Greeks called **POLTOS**, and the Romans **PULS**, and hcncc pulsc crop.

Both the Greeks and Romans had mixed feelings about the plant.

Greek seers and oracles refused to eat them, fearing it would interfere with their prophetic visions. Pythagoras, the famed Greek philosopher, was killed by enraged folks of Crotonia, when he could not cross a bean field in order to escape. Many of his disciples were killed shortly afterwards by soldiers of Dionysus, who ambushed them in a bean field.

Pythagoras probably instituted the ban on faba because he observed the consequences of favism. To him and his disciples, eating beans implied devouring one's own parents, causing serious disruption in the cycle of reincarnation.

The Roman Pliny believed that the souls of the dead were contained in the beans. Ceres, the Roman Goddess of Grain, is said to have refused to include them as gifts to man because they beclouded the second sight of her priest. Ovid said that witches put beans in their mouth when calling up spirits.

The Roman scholar, Diogenes Laertius wrote: "One should abstain from eating beans because they are full of the material which contains the largest portion of that animated matter of which our souls are made."

The Greek word for soul is **ANEMOS**, which also means wind. When eaten and processed in the human intestine, soul winds are released, and eager to resume their ascension to heaven, headed straight for the nearest opening, exiting with a cry of joy.

The Romans ate broad beans at funerals.

If all of this sounds strange, keep in mind that only recently has modern medical immunology recognized that genetically prone individuals of Mediterranean ancestry react to a substance in the beans that causes fatal dissolution of red blood cells, or favism.

When the Romans were Christianized, beans were thrown at ghosts on All Saint's Eve, our Halloween, and women would abstain from eating them for fear of being impregnated by the ghosts of frustrated men.

Some individuals are so sensitive and allergic that they faint at the scent of the flower blossoms. Symptoms of favism can occur after inhaling the pollen, in sensitive individuals.

The scent is persistent and widespread, reminiscent of honey and auratum lily. In Suffolk, England, the scent was believed helpful to children suffering whooping cough. In some areas of England, the scent was considered a powerful aphrodisiac. Ancient Celts applied the name beano to a funeral bean feast.

Miners in Suffolk thought more mine accidents occurred during its time of flowering.

Two conjugates of jasmonic acid with tyrosine, dopa, and dopamine links may explain, in part, the observed benefits.

Hildegard de Bingen, the 12th century abbess, suggested "there is not much harm if sick people eat Faba beans, since they do not produce as much mucous as peas."

The Brothers Grimm tale of Jack and the Beanstalk is undoubtedly a broad bean vine.

When I lived on the shores of Lesser Slave Lake, I grew Windsor Beans as a source of winter food. The pods were huge, up to a foot long, with furry insides protecting the large, flat, kidney shaped bean.

The seeds are edible while green (like fresh peas), as well as the brown dried, after prolonged cooking (see below). The plants are nitrogen fixers, as are all legumes, and can be used as green manure.

Dr. King says that the stalks and husks when calcined and digested in white wine, are a good diuretic. The flowers, as an infusion, are reputed effective in gout and gravel. The bean flour has long been used in Europe as a remedy for diarrhea.

Fava beans are a staple in some Middle Eastern countries. They are dried and ground into flour, but more often cooked in a sauce. They were quite popular in colonial America, with fourteen varieties available from one Philadelphia seed man in 1803.

When introduced to northern Alberta, the Cree named it **MISTATIMOPEN-SAK**, or **KISTIKANIS**, meaning Horse Bean.

In the American southwest the beans are browned in the oven, decocted with a little salt and taken as a soup to prevent pneumonia or cold lungs. If pneumonia is already present, a paste is prepared from the ground dry beans with hot water, and applied three times daily to the chest and back.

The flour is often combined with rye or spelt flour to make flat breads. In France today, faba flour is added at 2% or less to give baguettes their distinct aroma, add flavour to the bread, boost the rising process and whiten the crumb of breads made with less refined flours.

In Asia, they are fermented into a shoyu-like (soy) sauce or sprouted as a green edible. In India, the seeds are roasted and eaten like peanuts, while in China the re-hydrated beans are steamed and served cold in sesame oil dressing.

They are sometimes sprouted and cooked as a stir-fry or added to soups.

The shoots are boiled in oil and salt and used to rouse drunkards from their stupor in parts of China.

They have also been used as meat extenders or substitutes, as well as a skim milk substitute.

A tofu-like product has been developed, from faba beans, by Zee et al, at Laval University in Quebec. A decantation process was used with details available in *Canadian Institutional Food Science Technology* 1987 20:4.

In certain people, an inherited form of anemia can take place when the beans are eaten in large quantities over extended time, especially raw. They are toxic only to those lacking a digestive enzyme, which normally destroys the hemolytic aspect of the seed. The substances responsible are vicine and convicine, with their oxidized forms reacting with glutathione. Young boys, especially of the eastern Mediterranean and parts of China have this congenital G6PD (glucose phosphate dehydrogenase) deficiency.

The leaves are edible when cooked, or lightly steamed.

Broad bean flowers were traditionally used in the treatment of coughs, as well as uro-genital complaints, including difficulty with urination. Externally, the flowers were poulticed for skin inflammation, warts and burns, while the dry powdered bean helped heal mouth sores.

In ancient Egypt, faba beans were used as an ingredient in mouth rinses, for dressings, and in applications to "soften" stiff limbs. The bean meal was made into a paste with oil and honey, and applied to prolapsed rectums.

A modern Italian slang word for female genitals is **FAVA**, meaning bean.

In Scotland, the witches did not fly on conventional broomsticks, but used faba bean stalks instead. The pod fluff was used traditionally to remove warts, soothe chapped lips and remove the sting of nettles.

Fava Bean is originally from Western Asia and North Africa, and now grown in North America. In 1998, just over 247 tonnes of faba beans were produced commercially in Alberta, for a value of $113,000. In neighboring Saskatchewan, just over 2,000 acres were seeded, averaging 550 kilos per acre yield, or about 30 bushels to the acre. Seeding rate is three bushels to the acre.

They should be planted early as they require about 115 frost free days to mature, and can take a spring frost much better than one in the fall.

St. Denis Seed Farms near St. Albert has been growing faba for a number of years, including a white variety "Snowbird" with zero tannins. Lack of these compounds may help promote more use in livestock feed including hogs. Up to 35% faba can be added to pig rations; and would give prairie producers a replacement for soy meal at very competitive prices.

Another interesting form is the Tick Bean, in reference to the tan coloured, small seed, with a distinct nutty flavour.

In French, it is known as **FEVE À COUPER**, meaning "snipping" fava, in reference to the large floppy leaf buds used as a potherb. The flowers are sweet and fragrant, and the pod production higher than most other fava.

When the top buds are picked as salad greens, the plant sets pods more quickly.

Another favourite of mine is Crimson Flowering Fava, with edible green beans, flowers and leaves. The flowers of this two foot tall Fava are intensely magenta.

The straw of broad beans burned to ash can be mixed into top soil, and quickens the germination of parsley seeds.

Intercropping faba beans with Coriander gives a good yield advantage. Biennial caraway is another good option.

Various species of *Polygonum* genus including Bistort, Knotweed, Water Smartweed and Lady's Thumb produce water extracts effective at controlling *Aphis fabae*.

Ants collect nectar from the leaf nectaries at the bracts. The plants benefit as the ants keep caterpillars away.

Faba bean tolerates petroleum pollution up to 10% crude oil/sand w/w in work by Radwan et al, *Int J Phytoremed* 2000 2 suggesting use in contaminated oil and gas well sites.

American Vetch is a native vine-like legume very common to open woods, with white flowers, and small pods. The young shoots were cooked as greens by various Native tribes.

The Iroquois decocted the roots as a love medicine. The Navaho smudged the plant near horses to increase their endurance; and infusion of the plant as an eyewash.

The Squaxin tribe made an infusion of the crushed leaves as a bath for relieving soreness.

One magical use of vetch roots is for fidelity. If your love one has gone astray, rub the root of the vetch on your body and then wrap it in cloth and place it under your pillow. This will remind them that you're still around, waiting.

American Vetch is promoted, by Alberta Research Council in Vegreville, as a native reclamation plant. The seed weight is 60-80 thousand per kilo, with a seeding rate of 100-150 seeds per metre row. You can expect a 78% germination rate in 3-7 days with scarification; 75% in 14 days without.

The forage is palatable to livestock, particularly sheep, and browsed by mule deer

Studies on ecdysterone (see Maral Root) administration to faba leaves at a low concentration of 30 ppm, promotes accumulation of photosynthetic products without any effect on the rate of respiration.

Tufted Vetch is an introduced perennial with purplish, blue flowers and a weak, sprawling stem. It was originally brought to North America as a fodder or green manure, that has escaped and flourished. The plant has come to symbolize reason, and dedicated to the birth date, November 24th.

The young shoots, leaves, pods and seeds are all edible after proper identification and cooking. Studies conducted in Northern Ontario and Quebec, found no increase in body weight of sheep after 3 weeks, and a loss in steers after four. The protein content and coefficient of digestibility are high, but the coefficient of cellulose is low.

The unripe seeds look like small peas, but contain traces of hydrocyanic acid, that is removed by cooking. The ripe seeds can also be sprouted. Tufted vetch contains pyrimidin derivatives that cause photosensitivity illness.

Russell Willier, noted Cree healer, uses the roots in combinations for heart and stomach cramps. He calls the plant **PIMAHOPOKWA**, or climbing vine.

Two patents exist for *F. cracca*. One is for the lectins potential as an anti-retroviral drug; the other using affinity absorbents for isolating lectins. One chain lectins are specific to blood type A.

The plant contains 19 phenolic compounds, nine flavonoids as well as quercetin, kaempferol, apigenin and disometin.

Woolly Vetch is an introduced annual found in the southern part of our region. It is grown mainly to increase the nitrogen content of the soil.

As a winter annual, it is often a contaminant in fall-sown rye. Several reports indicate grazing on *V. villosa* has caused diarrhea, dermatitis, and conjunctivitis, and sexual excitement in cattle. Hair vetch poisoning can have a high mortality rate.

Beta cyano-L-alanine, implicated in locoweed toxicity, is present in the seeds of *V. villosa*. The blue flowers contain interesting anthocyanins.

Woolly Vetch is capable of detecting the smallest intensity of light. A 25 watt lamp in clear air and complete darkness can be detected and located by the seedling tips at a distance of 19 miles; a 100 watt lamp at 44 miles. For a plant without a telescope this is truly remarkable.

Two plant physiologists in the United States have found that annual vetch works very well as an organic mulch to replace plastic sheeting in growing tomatoes; as well as other row crops like snap beans, peppers, eggplants and cantaloupe.

The annual vetch is seeded in newly plowed and disked fields about two months before winter freeze up.

They become dormant but in spring they begin to grow again vigorously. The day before planting your tomatoes, mow the vetch with a high-speed flail mower and leave the residue on beds. Transplant the young tomato plants right through the mulch, into the soil. The killed vetch forms an organic blanket that feeds nitrogen and other nutrients into the soil.

When hairy vetch and turnips are planted together, the turnip greens are aphid free, due to the vetch providing shelter for ladybugs that love to eat aphids.

Work by Fujihara et al, in Japan, showed hairy vetch mulch resulted in a 60-80% reduction of weed biomass. Even more effective was to cover the row with the aerial parts of living hairy vetch; especially for root crops.

In parts of France, the seeds of *V. sativa* were traditionally used in soup and flour for bread. Work by Han et al, *Biotech Lett* 28(23) identified a means of producing R-cyanohydins from the seeds.

MEDICINAL

CONSTITUENTS *V. cracca* -leaves- kaempferol-3-0-rhamnoside, proanthocyanidins, one chain lectins. The seed lectin of F. cracca is specific for human blood type A.
V. villosa- flowers- contain the 3-O-alpha-rhamnopyranoside-5-O-beta glucopyranosides of petunidin (71%), delphinidin (12%), and malvidin (9%)
Aerial parts- cyanamide
V. faba pods- five flavonoid aglycons and 8 flavonol glycosides. As the colour of the pod changes from green to reddish and finally dark brown, the flavanoids increase; and then decrease at full maturity.
seeds- 11.4 mcg/kg of estradiol monobenzoate from green seeds, including genistein, daidzein and formomonetin; wyerone, medicarpin, and epoxide (phytoalexins); vicine (vicioside, 0.4-0.8%), convicine (0.1-0.6%), isolectins-favine-L-3.4-dihydroxyphenylalanine (L-dopa, up to 8%), tannins, starch.
sprouted seed- amylase and vitamin C activity maximum on third day.
Protein- green, 5.2%; dry 25%. Plant also contains convicine, wyerone epoxide, medicarpin, and gibberillin A-53, as well as jasmonic and isojasmonic acids.
stem- genistein and daidzein

Faba beans contain natural L-dopa which penetrates the intestinal epithelial cells and is transported through the blood stream to the brain capillaries where it is converted into dopamine.

The beans should be eaten, when not fully mature, but when young, with a thin skin and easy to digest. Up to 90% of patients afflicted with Parkinson's disease at an early age respond quickly.

It is easily oxidized two to three days after harvest and vanishes completely as the plant stops growing and begins to dry.

When sprouted, the L-dopa content increases ten times (10x), and is worth investigating as a potential commercial product.

Patient report a marked improvement each time they eat a meal of fresh Faba beans. A commercial product called Dopa Bean, is now available with standardized content of natural L-dopa from faba bean.

In a study by Rabey et al, *Advanced Neurology* 1993 60 six patients with Parkinson's disease were taken off their medications, and after 12 hours were given 250 grams of cooked faba beans. Significant improvements in motor symptoms were found, compared to those on 125 mg of L-DOPA, and 12.5 mg of carbidopa. Plasma levels of L-DOPA increased after faba ingestion in a manner comparable to oral administration of the drug, suggesting it was transported into the CNS and converted to dopamine. Work in England has found the highest concentrations of L-dopa in bean variety WH 305.

Researchers at the Prince of Wales Medical Research Institute in Sydney, Australia have found a new test that may detect initial signs of Parkinson's disease, 7-20 years before symptoms appear. The test looks for antibodies to neuromelanin, which is produced when dopamine sensitive nerve cells are in a degenerative state.

Large amounts of L-dopa may cause priapsim, a painful, persistent erection that is not necessarily related to sexual arousal. As Faba beans have a reputation as an aphrodisiac, they might contain that little extra L-dopa that gives a more sustained erection.

When combined with Puncture Vine, there is a synergistic effect that appears to increase the body's absorption of L-dopa.

As Faba beans increase the brain's production of dopamine, this, in turn will decrease prolactin that stimulates milk production. If breastfeeding, and milk flow is deficient, do not eat the beans. Work by Koreneva, *Probl Endokrinol* 1980 26:6 found L-Dopa effective in treating women suffering amenorrhea-galactorrhea syndrome.

The medicinal uses of L-Dopa are amazingly widespread with good clinical studies on bone fracture, myocardial infarction, depression, amblyopia, and optic neuropathy, measles encephalitis, male sterility, peptic ulcer, restless leg syndrome, sleep disorders and various forms of dystonia.

Faba may be useful in the treatment of epilepsy.

Work by Salih et al, *Epilepsy Behav* 2008 12:1 found evidence of binding to glycine receptors and anti-convulsant properties. A synergistic pattern with diazepam was noted in the study.

As an aside, it should be noted that fresh banana peels contain 6-12 microM per gram of dopamine. Could this be the source of Mellow Yellow during the 1960s, when smoking banana peels was touted as a way to get high? The banana fruit contains (-)-salsolinol, which shows dopamine antagonism *in vivo*.

Dopamine helps alleviate cravings associated with addictions like alcohol and nicotine.

An older study by Macarulla et al, in the *British Journal of Nutrition* 85:5 found that both the whole bean and the protein isolate from Faba were strongly anti-oxidative.

Okada et al, later confirmed the protein extract is water soluble. *J of Nutritional Science and Vitaminology* 2000 46:1.

In Traditional Chinese Medicine, faba bean is used for edema, in the form of a tea. It is most commonly called **CAN COU**, meaning silkworm bean, but is also known as **HU DOU**, foreign bean, **MA CHI DOU**, horse tooth bean, and **NAN DOU**, south bean.

The fresh beans can be crushed into a paste and applied externally to tinea capitis, while the mashed leaves help heal indolent leg ulcers.

When dry, the beans are ground into a powder. Two teaspoons are dissolved in warm water and taken three times daily for chronic diarrhea and bloody stools.

And the powder can be boiled with sugar to treat children with poor appetite and diarrhea; brown sugar with presence of blood from the anus. The older the powder, the stronger the effect.

One antacid product in health food stores contains faba bean flour for acid neutralizing effect.

The leaves can be juiced and 20 ml twice daily ingested for tuberculosis with coughing of blood.

The leaves, flowers, seeds and seed hull all possess anti-bacterial activity against *E. coli, Staphylococcus aureus, Shigella* species, *Bacillus subtilis, Serratia marcesens,* and *Micrococcus pyogenes*. Peyvast et al, *Pak J Bio Sci* 2007 10:3.

The seed coat extracted with methanol shows activity against *S. aureus, B. subtilis, B. cereus, E. coli, Candida albicans, C. maltosa* and *Cryptococcus neoformans*. Akroum et al, *Eur J Sci Res* 2009 31:2.

The aerial parts show antioxidant activity and inhibit topoisomerase I enzyme activity, suggestive of chemoprotective benefit. Spanou et al, *J Ag Food Chem* 2008 56.

The flowers combine well with corn silk in the treatment of hypertension, simmered and taken as a tea. When cooled, the flower tea helps ease the pain of kidney stones and sciatica, and stop bleeding.

The shells can be simmered and the water taken for dysuria, while the stems when decocted help resolve bloody diarrhea.

Nohara et al, from Kumamoto University, Japan studied the composition and hepatoprotective properties of Faba Bean. Typical oleanene glycosides with a methyl group at C28 and having the fabatriosyl moiety showed strong liver protective activity. *Studies in Plant Science* 1999 6:31.

Madar and Stark, in the *British Journal of Nutrition* 2002 88:3 mention faba beans lipid lowering effects and as a source of anti-oxidative and chemopreventative factors.

Sauer, in his Compendious Herbal, suggests Broad Bean flour for swellings of the bosoms, and "when the member swells so that one cannot urinate, as can easily happen to those afflicted by the stone when the stone settles in the duct, then cook some broad beans in milk to a porridge consistency. Apply this thick and warm around the member."

The stems contain isoflavones at the rate of over 1 gram/kilo, and due to the prodigious growth may have some future nutraceutical application.

The biochemical composition of faba beans cooked by different extrusion temperatures and feed moisture was examined by Prakrati et al, *J of Food Science and Tech Mysore*, 2000 37.

Cooking at 75 degrees C, increased tryptophan, methionone, and iron levels by 20%, and decreased both calcium and phosphorus.

Faba beans increase both sodium excretion and diuresis through renal dopamine receptors, according to work by Vered et al, *Planta Medica* 1997 63:3.

Wyerone derived from faba bean has anti-fungal properties.

Lectins from faba bean can alter the differentiation, adhesion and proliferation of colorectal cancer cells. Work by Jordinson et al, *Gut* 1999 44:5 found agglutinin from the bean stimulated an undifferentiated colon cancer cell line to differentiate into gland like structures, with the adhesion molecule epCAM involved. The authors suggest that dietary or therapeutic intake of faba bean lectins may slow the progression of colon cancer.

The roots are a narcotic poison. Wyeronic acid is formed when the plant is attacked by botrytis, and exhibits anti-fungal activity.

Tufted Vetch (*V. cracca*) leaves in water extract show activity against myco-bacteria. Two plant patents exist, one for its lectins, and their activity as an anti-retroviral drug. The lectin is blood group A specific. It accumulates cyanamide.

Woolly Vetch (*V. villosa*) seeds contain three alpha galactosides of D-pinitol. This compound, found in chickpea, lentil, and stressed pine needles, is gaining importance in the maintenance of blood sugar levels.

The plant also contains cyanamide, a plant growth inhibitor.

SEED OIL

CONSTITUENTS- composed mainly of oleic acid (57.5%) and linoleic acid (35%); with about 7.5% saturated fatty acids, mainly stearic acid.

HYDROSOL

The flowers and green pods are diuretic and sedative to the urinary tract. According to Culpepper, "water distilled from fresh husks drunk was effectual against the stone and to provoke urine.

Sauer wrote "several loths (2 loths- one ounce) of water of broad bean flowers drunk in the morning before breakfast will promote urine and drive out gravel".

FLOWER ESSENCES

Tufted Vetch (*V. cracca*) flower essence is the remedy for many cases of sexual difficulty. Male or female, the difficulties are often caused by a totally incorrect "self-image".

For many there is an inability to come "up-front", and accept the sexual aspect of their nature. The roots of these difficulties are nearly always in childhood, and are frequently due to heavy conditioning. There is also an inability to see the games that one plays on the sexual level, and a tendency to always blame the other sex when things do not turn out as the person would have wished. **BAILEY**

Vetch (*Vicia* sp.) flower essence helps to build healthy boundaries among members of a community, allowance for others' differences and to help teamwork and working together. **HUMMINGBIRD**

Fava (*Vicia faba*) essence facilitates all functions of brain activity, including memory, energy and sense of well being. It is useful for balancing hormones. Strength, energy and radiant vitality come from being in balance. Good for menopause, supports a parasitic cleanse.
STAR PERUVIAN

Tufted Vetch essence helps develop independence and self-confidence.
CHOMING

Tufted Vetch essence strengthens self- determination and realization, helps one feel clear and free of compulsive acts and dependencies.
MARIANA

PERSONALITY TRAITS

Tufted Vetch
I am one of those rather entangling weeds
Who makes good use of my neighbours I fear.
And I go through your garden, leaving my seeds
To make sure I come back the following year. **CAMERON**

"I remember once being in the train beside the open window; I was reading and quite absorbed in a very interesting book; presently I became aware that my heart was beating and I had my 'beanfield (faba bean) feeling'.

I was just saying to myself, 'This book is as exciting as a beanfield', when I looked out of the window and saw we were passing a beanfield! The effect passed off as soon as we were out of the scent zone, which proved it was not the book. It was a most delightful sensation, and the excitement pleasurable; a sort of happy, buoyant ecstasy." **F. A. HAMPTON**

SPIRITUAL PROPERTIES

Mojo beans are seen as a profound blessing from God. In Catholicism, they are associated with St. Joseph's Day and are placed on the altar. During one of Sicily's severe famines, the people prayed to St. Joseph to be delivered from the crisis. As a result of their prayers, the Mojo beans thrived while other crops failed. They became a symbol of abundance and prosperity. **S. GREGG**

OTHER PROPERTIES

Lima Beans, like their cousin Faba, have been found to be good communicators, according to new research from Japan.

Like some other plants, Lima can let its neighbors know when attacked by a pest like the spider mite.

The munching releases volatile compounds that are carried through the air to neighboring plants, which then prepare chemical defenses against infestation.

This has been known for some time, but in early 2000, researchers reporting in *Nature*, discovered the volatile compounds that activate five defense genes in an un-infested plant.

The plants were also found to differentiate between a mite infestation and physical damage from say, stepping on the plant. These compounds were ignored by neighboring plants.

Fabaceae is the longest English word that can also be a hexadecimal numeral (consisting only of a, b, c, d, e and f). This is an old system created in the 1950s for computer ASCII code.

RECIPES

DOPA BEAN- One or two capsules daily of standardized faba bean extract.

A rapid reversed phase HPLC method derived by Perumal and Becker, *Food Chemistry* 2001 72:3 may prove useful in determining L-dopa percentage in beans. The variety WH305 appears to contain the highest % of L-dopa.

COOKED FABA BEANS- Usually broad beans require soaking overnight and cooking the hydrated beans for about two hours. A quick method involves blanching for seven minutes in boiling water, followed by hydration in a soaking medium of sodium bicarbonate, sodium carbonate and trisodium phosphate and cooking in 2.5% brine. The cooking time is reduced to fifteen, with good flavour and free from lipoxygenase, hemagglutinin and trypsin inhibitor activity.

CAUTION- Favism is a hemolytic anemia disease occurring in individuals suffering from a blood enzyme deficiency, glucose-6-phosphate de-hydrogenase (G6PD), that can be fatal in infants. The deficiency occurs almost exclusively in populations living around the Mediterranean, but today affects about 400 million people worldwide.

It is believed caused by the presence of faba beans, especially green pods and seeds, of two glycosidic pyrimidine derivatives, vicine and convicine, and/or their hydrolytic products (aglycones) divicine and isouramil. Some sensitive individuals react to the pollen. Jaundice can be one symptom that is more obvious.

It is believed a trade off for malaria resistance, as this condition produces red blood cells that starve the malaria parasite of oxygen. Or, more accurately, G6PD deficient red blood cells contain too little of a metabolite essential for the survival of the parasite.

Ironically, all known anti-malarial drugs are contraindicated for these individuals.

The gene for G6PD enzyme is carried on the X chromosome, so males are more likely to be afflicted. For a female to have the condition, genes on both of her X chromosomes would have to be affected.

Morel mushrooms should be avoided, for same reasons, by same faba bean sensitive individuals.

GINKGO
MAIDENHAIR TREE
(*Ginkgo biloba* L.)

PARTS USED- leaf, seeds

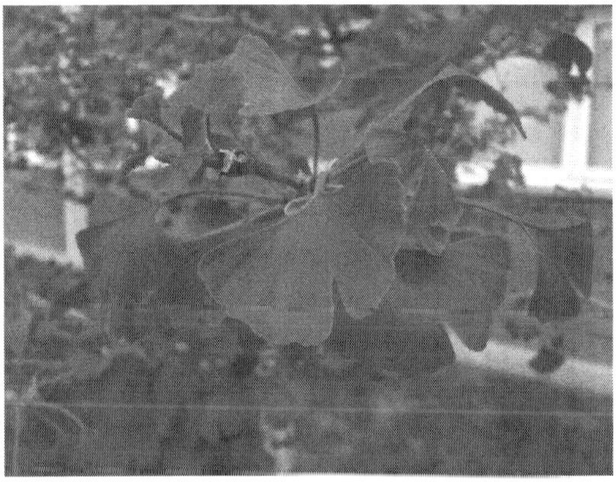

Ginko leaves

Ginkgo is one of our oldest living species of tree, dating back over 225 million years. It is almost extinct in the wild and now widely cultivated. It is revered for its longevity, as suggested by the Chinese colloquial name **KUNG SUN SHU** meaning, grandfather and grandson tree. Other names include Ancestor tree, Buddha's Fingernail Tree and Eyes of the Cosmic Spirit Tree. In ancient China, it was called I-cho (duck's foot tree).

The oldest known specimen Li Jiawan Grand Ginkgo King, is found near Guiyang, the capital of Guizhou province. It is three thousand years old, 30 meters tall and measures 15.6 meters in girth at breast height. In China and Korea, the plant is revered by Buddhists and planted as temple tree. In Japan, followers of Shinto do the same.

Ginkgo is from the Japanese and may derived from the Chinese ideogram pronounced Yin- Kuo, meaning "silver fruit".

It is mentioned briefly in TCM during the Ming dynasty in 1436 AD, but really did not become a well-known medicinal until the latter half of 20th century. The name Maidenhair is related to the similarity of leaf to the fern. In fact, many scientists believe it may be the first tree to evolve. At least four different species of Ginkgo shared the planet with dinosaurs, making it a true living fossil.

It is possible that it is the first tree to arise from prehistoric landscapes and tower over tree ferns and cycads, the ancient palm-like plants. Fossil records show it was once widespread throughout the planet, from China to California and from Europe to the island of Spitsbergen in the Arctic Circle.

It is a slow growing tree that can survive in the cold, dry climate of my native Alberta. In warmer climates it is an urban tree that can resist disease, insects and pollution. The bark sap is said to act as a fire retardant.

It is said that one ginkgo tree near ground zero of the 1945 Hiroshima nuclear bomb blast, sprouted green leaves a few months after the explosion.

The fresh seeds are used in Asian tradition, but are potentially poisonous. I have seen them widely available in Chinese food stores, but extreme caution is advised. The red-dyed fruits are often consumed at Chinese weddings.

The Japanese call the downward growing aerial roots **CHICHI** meaning, nipple or breast. One ginkgo in Sendai City is planted over the grave of Emporer Shoumu's wet nurse. She vowed to Buddha that she would give milk to all the women who had none. The tree is over 1300 years old, and women who cannot produce breast milk pray at the tree.

Topknot hair worn by Japanese men was called icho or ginkgo, due to the shape. The size, shape and position of the topknot showed social status, ranging from big ginkgo for samuri and sumo wrestlers to small ginkgo for merchants. Large ginkgo-leaf shaped topknots are still worn today by wrestlers to protect from head injury.

The method of reproduction is most unusual. In 1896, a Japanese botanist Sakugoro Hirase noticed the presence of motile sperm swimming toward the waiting egg cells. Motile sperm was at that time considered associated with primitive non-seed plants such as moss and ferns, again suggesting the relationship to these ancient plants.

The use of ginkgo leaves for medicinal purpose began in Germany, with one particular extract (EGb 761) widely tested, prescribed and used throughout Europe.

When first introduced in European monasteries, it was used to eliminate frequent urination during times of worship.

The pinkish-yellow fruit hang in pairs and have an unpleasant smell. They attract, in the wild, leopards and civets that feed on them at night.

The seeds need to pass through the gut to improve germination by up to 71%.

MEDICINAL

CONSTITUENTS- leaf- ginkgolides A, B, C, M, terpenes (bilobalides), flavonoids including ginkgetin, quercitin, kaempferol, apigenin, proanthocyanidins, ginkgolic acid, kynurenic acid.
Seed and seed coat- alkaloids including ginkgotoxic (4-methoxylpyridoxine), cyanogenic glycosides, urushiol (found in poison ivy), anacardic acid, histidine and fatty acids including butyric, caproic, caprylic, hexanoic, linoleic and palmitic acids.

The active ingredients in the leaf are ginkgolides and the sesquiterpene bilobalide usually standardized to 24/6.

The ginkgolides, particularly ginkgolide B inhibit platelet activating factor (PAF) and 3'5'-cyclic GMP phosphodiesterase, that relaxes endothelium. The flavonoid fraction particularly quercitin, increases serotonin release and uptake, inhibits age-related reduction of muscarinergic cholinoceptors and alpha-adrenoceptors, and stimulates choline uptake in the hippocampus. Hundreds of studies have been conducted and a few of the more recent ones are cited here.

Eighteen studies involving 1672 patients support the use of ginkgo to treat dementia due to cardiovascular insufficiency.

A Cochrane review of 33 trials found "promising evidence of improvement in cognition and function. Birks et al, *The Cochrane Library* 2002 4

A systematic review and met-analysis looked at nine trials with 2372 patients, found ginkgo more effective than placebo for dementia and Alzheimer's disease.

In a 24 week clinical trial of 410 outpatients with mild to moderate dementia, ginkgo helped alleviate behavioral and neuropsychiatric symptoms, and improved the well being of caregivers as well. Bachinskaya N et al, *Neuropsychiatr Dis Treat* 2011 7 209-15.

A twenty-year study followed 3612 non dementia patients and found cognitive decline was lower in subjects taking ginkgo biloba extract. The nootropic medication, piracetam, did not show this effect. Amieva H et al, *PLoS One* 2013 8:1.

A combination of ginkgo and bacopa showed improvement in memory and attention in young adults. Das A et al, *Pharmacol Biochem Behav* 2002 73:4.

The herb is approved in Germany for the treatment of cerebral insufficiency (senile dementia), tinnitus, vertigo and intermittent claudication, or poor circulation to the lower legs. In fact, ginkgo is a peripheral circulatory stimulant, allowing increased blood flow to the extremities of the body including the brain, hands, feet and even genital organs.

One study by Brown et al, found increased alpha wave brain activity and decreased theta wave activity. *Q Rev Nat Med* 1997 summer 91-6.

Gingko extracts may be useful in blood sugar dysregulation. A three month study found the herb increases pancreatic beta cell function with increased insulin and C-peptide levels. Kudolo GB, *J Clin Pharmacol* 2000 40 647-54. A more recent systematic review of 16 trials suggests it may help in treating early diabetic neuropathy. Zhang Lei et al, *Evid Based Complement Altern Med* 2013 February 24.

Chronic elevation of blood sugar can activate cardiovascular inflammation and increased endothelial adhesion leading to atherogenesis. Ginkgo biloba reduced this inflammation by inhibition of interleukin-6. Chen JS et al, *Cardiovas Diabetol* 2012 11-49.

Ginkgo is almost a specific for tinnitus. A recent systematic review of eight R PC trials by Alexander von Boetticher suggests standardized EGb 761 extract is an evidence-based treatment option for tinnitus.

The chemotherapy drug cisplatin induces significant hearing loss and balance problems. A combination of ginkgo biloba and cilostazol may reduce hearing loss and dizziness without interfering with drug treatment. Tian CJ et al, *Cell Death Dis* 2013 4:2.

Many years ago I developed a line of herbal supplements for femMed. Libido was created to enhance sexual desire and includes ginkgo to increase blood flow to genital region by relaxing smooth muscle via nitric oxide influence.

A study of 68 women taking ginkgo for eight weeks with sex therapy, enhanced orgasm function compared with placebo. Meston CM et al, *Arch Sex Behav* 2008 37:4 530-47.

The herb has shown to potentiate papaverine in men suffering erectile dysfunction. Sikora R et al, *J Urol* 1989 141:188A.

It also showed benefit in anti-depressant induced sexual dysfunction. Cohen AJ et al, *J Sex Marital Ther* 1998 24:2 139-43. This includes SSRIs, MAOIs and tricyclic medications. Ginkgo may help glaucoma. In a randomized trial of 30 patients with normal tension glaucoma, the herb increased ocular blood flow, volume and velocity compared to placebo. Park JW et al, *Korean J Opthalmol* 2011 25:5 323-8.

Twenty-one patients with normal tension glaucoma were followed for over twelve years. Gingko biloba at 80 mg twice daily slowed progression of visual field damage especially in zone 1 corresponding to the superior central field. Lee J et al, *J Glaucoma* 2013 22(9): 780-4.

A systematic review and meta-analysis suggests efficacy for patients with dementia and as an adjunct for chronic schizophrenia. Brondino N et al, *Evid Based Compl Altern Med* 2013;2013:1-11.

Ginkgo leaf is rarely thought of as anti-viral, but one study suggests activity against influenza A (H1N1 and H3N2) and influenza B viruses. Haruyama T & Nagata K. *Journal Natural Medicine* 2013 67(3):636-42.

I have used ginkgo extracts successfully in treatment of childhood asthma.

Ginkgo seeds, dried and processed, with the external seed coat and fleshy pulp removed, are used in TCM for treatment of lung problems including tuberculosis, bronchitis and asthma. The fresh seeds are neuro-toxic. Ginkgotoxin is a competitive antagonist of B6 and inhibits GABA formation. If levels of GABA fall, neuronal activity increases and epileptic seizure may occur.

In Korea, the fruit is used for coughs, astma and bladder complaints.

HOMEOPATHY

Tired, can't think, poor concentration, brain fog, aversion to company, wants to left alone. Apathetic, emotional numbness, distracted, time distortion, inflexible.

Dreams of danger and disaster involving water, earthquakes, explosions, death in family, and misfortune. Cold hands and feet, dry skin. Irrational fears with rapid speech.

Sensations as if skull too small, brain falling apart, legs heavy or made of rubber. Headaches, tinnitus and vertigo. Clenching of right hand with trembling. Insomnia between 2 and 3 am. Nightmares with dreams of corpses.

Aggravation from cold or walking, from drinking or from looking up and to the right. Better from heat and rest.

DOSE- Mother tincture to 30X. Proving by Maury with seven provers and mother tincture, and two provers with 6C in 1933. Self-experimentation by McIvor at 6X for ten weeks in 1971. Proving by Swoboda & Konig with 25 volunteers at 30X in 1987 and another 25 in 1989. Proving by Anne Schadde with sixteen provers at 30C 1995-96.

All provings were made with parts of the plant without seed. The mother tincture is made from fresh leaves gathered in spring.

LEAF ESSENCE

Maidenhair Tree releases the pattern of being insufficiently considerate of others in interpersonal relationships. This results in empathy and a clear appreciation of others' feelings and perspective.

FALLING LEAF ESSENCES

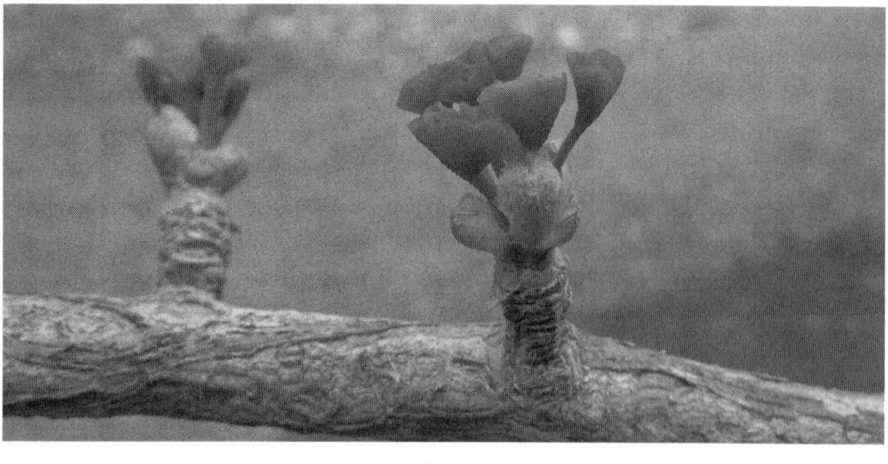

Young Ginko leaves

BOTANICA POETICA
Ginkgo biloba
Forgetting where you put the key
Or, what you ate for snack?
The issue is your memory
You'd like to get that back
Here's an ancient Chinese tree
The leaves affect the brain
An extract for the elderly
More facts they will retain
Improve cerebral circulation
A neuropathic gift
Enhance a sexual situation
When the penis needs a lift
And if your feet are cold
The circulation is too slow
Ginkgo Biloba, it is told
Improves the blood to flow
If your ears are ringing
You've tinnitus or vertigo
You're getting very frustrated…
This calls for some Ginkgo!
The benefits may take some time
So take it in full swing
Remember to take your Ginkgo
You might remember everything!
SYLVIA CHATROUX MD

RECIPES

STANDARDIZED EXTRACT (24/6) 50:1- This is only product you want to use. It is standardized to 24% ginkgo flavonol glycosides and 6% terpene lactones of which 2.9% is bilobalide and 3.1% is ginkgolides A, B, and C.

DOSE- 120-240 mg daily unless otherwise advised.

CAUTION- Fifteen published case reports describe the use of ginkgo and a bleeding event. Most involved serious medical conditions including 8 cases of intracranial bleeding. Thirteen of the 15 cases identified other risk factors for bleeding. Only six reported that when ginkgo was stopped, bleeding did not recur. Bent S et al, *J Gen Intern Med* 2005 20:7.

A one year study of 309 patients taking Coumadin or aspirin with the herb reported one stroke and one subdural hematoma, both in placebo group. Le Bars PL et al, *JAMA* 1997 278:16. A randomize DB PC crossover study of outpatients on stable long-term warfarin found no change with addition of ginkgo or CoQ10. Engelsen J et al, *Ugeskr Laeger* 2003 165:18.

However, it may be best to avoid any blood thinners, anti-platelets including aspirin and concurrent use of Ginkgo biloba. Also discontinue use for two weeks before surgery.

The literature cites a number of positive herb-drug interactions. Combined with trimipramine in eight patients with major depression for four weeks, sleep patterns improved. When ginkgo supplementation was stopped, the effects were reversed.

When taken with haloperidol for schiophrenia, it increased effectiveness of drug and reduced the extrapyramidal side effect. Immune function also improved. See *Herbal Contraindications and Drug Interactions plus Herbal Adjuncts with Medicines* 4th Ed by Francis Brinker for up to date information.

GOTU KOLA
BRAHMI
INDIAN PENNYWORT
(*Centella asiatica* [L.] Urban.)
(*Hydrocotyle asiatica* L.)
PARTS USED- aerial

Gotu Kola is derived from the Sinhala name for the plant. Brahmi related to the development of Brahman, the Supreme Reality, helping to strengthen nervous function and promote longevity, intelligence and memory.

Gotu Kola is a slender, creeping perennial with long stems that will root at the nodes.

It is eaten as a green vegetable throughout India and southeast Asia.

Apparently, it is relished by elephants in Sri Lanka. And they have good memories!

It is considered an Araliaceous hydrocotyloid, and although a member of the Apiaceae family, it has many botanical and therapeutic similarities to the Aralia genus.

Fresh juice, or fresh plant tinctures are best.

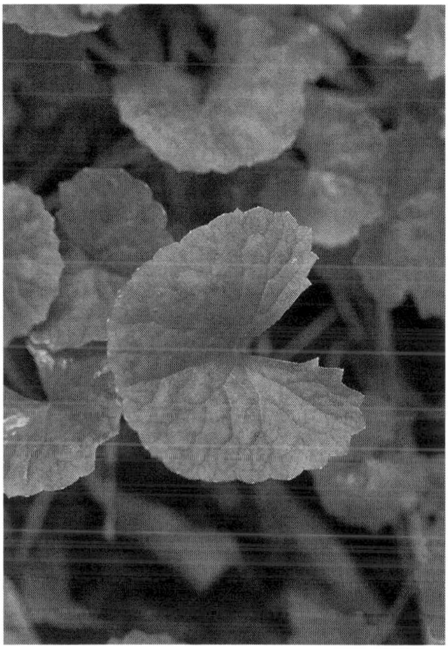

Gotu Kola leaves

MEDICINAL

CONSTITUENTS- various triterpenoids including asiaticoside A & B, madecassoside, braminoside, brahmoside, brahminoside, thankuniside, isothankunoside; triterpene acis like Asiatic acid, 6-hydroxy Asiatic acid, madecassic acid, madasiatic acid, brahmic acid, isobrahmic acid, betulinic acid and isothankuic acid, flavones including quercitin, kaempferol and astragalin, alkaloid hydrocotylin, tannins, amino acids, essential oils, vitamin B complex and resins.

Gotu Kola is most well-known for its ability to improve memory. A number of human studies on both children and the elderly suggest that more attention be paid to this remarkable herb for treatment of senile dementia and Alzheimer's disease.

The herb has been found in studies by Chatterjee et al 1992, to increase brain GABA levels. Other studies have found water extracts given to animals reduce anxiety levels in a manner similar to diazepam.

In a group of mentally-challenged children given either 500 mg of dried whole plant powser in capsules or placebo, intelligence quotient tests found, after three month, those taking the herb showed significant improvement in memory, concentration, attention, vocabulary and social cooperation and adjustment. Appa Rao et al, *J Res Ind Med* 1973 8:4 9-15.

A randomized, double-blind, placebo-controlled study of 28 senior citizens found 750 mg of herb taken one daily for two months enhanced working memory and improved self-rated mood. Wattanathorn J et al, *J Ethnopharm* 2008 116:2 325-32.

The exact mode of action has not been determined but neuro protection may be related to enzyme inhibition, prevention of amyloid plaque formation leading to Alzheimer's disease, prevention of dopamine neurotoxicity in Parkinson's disease and decreased oxidative stress. Orhan IE, *Evid Based Complement Altern Med* 2012 May 14.

Gotu Kola also improves physical performance in the elderly. In a study by Mato L et al, *Evid Based Complement Altern Med* 2011 June 7, eighty healthy volunteer received placebo or standardized extract of herb once daily for 90 days. Improvement of strength in lower extremities was confirmed in this DB, PC randomized trial.

Chronic venous insufficiency was noted in a systematic review of eight studies. Significant improvement in signs such as leg heaviness, pain and edema were noted. Chong NJ & Aziz Z, *Evid Based Complement Altern Med* 2013 February 21.

Diabetic neuropathy may also benefit. Compared to placebo, an extract from Idena called CAST improved subjective symptoms and prevented deterioration in an objective measure of nerve conduction. Although only 33 patients were involved, the randomized PC, DB study suggests Gotu Kola is safe, and effective for this growing epidemic. Soumyanath et al, *BMC Complement Altern Med* 2012 June 12.

Gotu Kola is used in a wide variety of inflammatory skin conditions including eczema, atopic dermatitis, varicose ulcers, psoriasis, lupus, leprosy and scleroderma. It combines well with Yellow Dock.

Todd Caldecott, note herbalist, suggests it can be used with Echinacea or Goldenseal in the treatment of infectious conditions, and with comfrey for wounds. Combine with Astragalus root for immune deficient conditions.

During my years of clinical practice, I had good success in a case of scleroderma in an elderly women using both internal standardized capsules and external application of a highly diluted gotu kola essential oil. See below.

The herb has an intelligence for helping the body find new vein pathways that have been blocked by surgery or mechanical injury.

It seems to assist in creating modulating collagen and glycosaminoglycan production and preventing keloid tissue from forming on recent wounds.

Asiatic acid, madecassic acid and asiaticoside have been found clinically effective on systemic scleroderma, abnormal scar formation and keloids. Hydrogels formed with a solubilizer like Na-DOC are most effective. Hong et al, *Arch Pharm Res* 2005 28:4.

Tablet, ointment and powdered forms were found efficacious in treatment of chronic and sub-chronic systemic scleroderma, as well as advanced focal scleroderma. Guseva et al, *Ter Arkh* 1998 70:5 58-61.

A methanol extract induced apoptosis in human breast cancer cell line MCF-7. Human implications are unknown.

The asiaticosides may raise blood sugar and cholesterol levels. Or do they? A recent study looked at a combination of this herb with *Andrographis paniculata* (see Immune). It was fed to rats on high fructose and fat diets and reseachers found a 70:30 ratio exhibited promising anti-diabetic effects. The effect was better than either herb individually. Nugroho AE et al, *Indian J Exp Biol* 2013 51:12.

HOMEOPATHY

Inclination for solitute, misanthropy and indifference. Dreams of being asleep. Disinclined to work, anorexia, aversion to smoking, weight in prostate and uterus. Blowing sound in ears, vertigo with heaviness of head, worse from standing.

Occiput sensitive to touch. Photophobia, upon opening eyes light trembles.

Frequent urge with burning sensation after urination. Unsteady or tottering gait.

DOSE- Mother tincture to 6th potency. Proving by Audouit with nine provers at tincture, third, fourth and sixth dilutions in 1856. Devergie observed effect of extract on leprosy in 1850s. Cazenave also observed extract effect on skin. He also described first case of lupus erythematosus in 1850. Observations by Ghose, Clark. Provings were done by the *Central Council for Research in Homeopathy* on 29 provers at tincture 6C and 200C between 1982-5.

ESSENTIAL OIL

Gotu Kola leaves and stems have been steam distilled and yield an oil with 41 identified compounds. Eighty percent are sesquiterpenes including 26.8% beta-caryophyllene, 33% alpha humulene and 10% germacrene D.

The essential oil is available but rarely found commercially. Most often it will be found in dilute form in almond carrier oil.

The oil, as 10% dilution, is very useful as external application in cases of scleroderma.

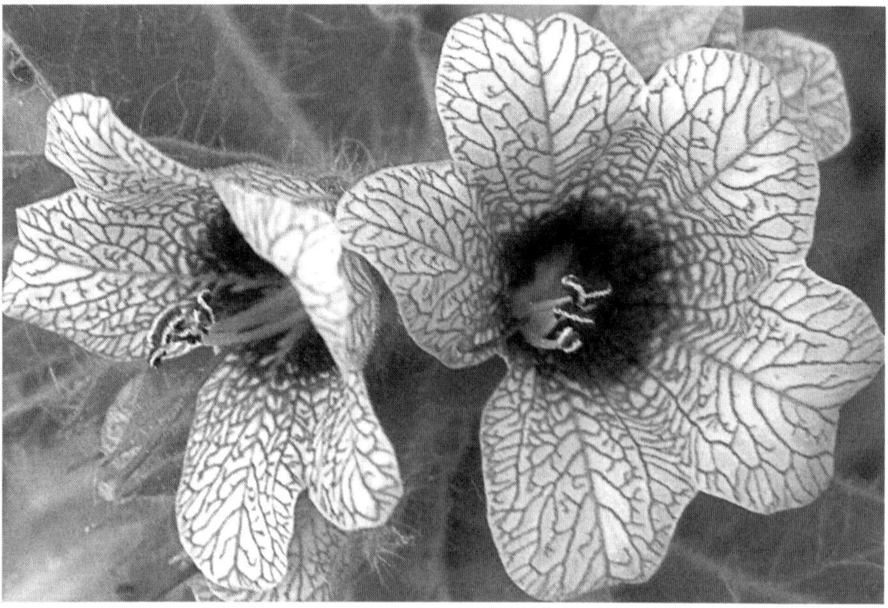

Henbane flowers

BOTANICA POETICA
Gotu Kola
Are you taking Calculus?
Need your brain cells to excel?
Want to boost your memory
This might prolong your life as well
Here we have of Tropic lands
For rapid growth of skin and hair
Speeds the healing of a wound
A salve to help your skin repair
Memory, intelligence
Gotu Kola, it can heal
Relieving stress, anxiety
Improve ability to deal
Here's a test that might impress
Feed this herb to your pet rats
He'll start to talk and win at chss
Tell me now, can you beat that?
Rejuvenate and stay young
Help damaged skin to improve
It's a tonic, helps fatigue
Put your life back in the groove!
SYLVIA CHATROUX MD

RECIPES

POWDER- 1-4 grams up to three times daily

TINCTURE- Thirty to sixty drops three times daily. Fresh plant tincture is made at 1:2 and 30% alcohol.

STANDARDIZED EXTRACT- 50 to 250 mg two to three times daily. Should contain 40% asiaticoside and other components listed.

CAUTION- Concurrent use with barbituates or benzodiazepines is not advised due to GABAnergic activity. It should not be used during pregnancy and caution is advised when patients are actively treating high cholesterol or blood sugar conditions. The herb may aggravate pruritis. Maybe.

BLACK HENBANE
(*Hyoscyamus niger* L.)
PARTS USED- whole plant, root

Were such things here as we do speak about?
Or have we eaten the insane root
That takes the reason prisoner? **SHAKESPEARE MACBETH**

Sleeping within mine orchard,
My custom always of the afternoon,
Upon my secure hour they uncle stole,
With juice of cursed **HEBENON** in a vial,
And in the porches of mine ear did pour the leprous distilment.
SHAKESPEARE

Henbane is the treasure flower of the Underworld. **M. MADEJSKY**

Presently he filled a cressat with firewood on which he strewed powdered henbane and, lighting it, went around the tent with it until the smoke entered the nostrils of the guards and they fell asleep, drowned by the drug. **1001 NIGHTS**

Henbane is from hennebone, which first appeared in the English language in 1398.

This, in turn, is derived from the much earlier **HENBELL** or **BELENE** from about 1000 AD; alluding to its bell-shaped calyx. More unlikely a source is Hen-killer, or Chicken killer, from the Anglo Saxon, **HENN** and **BANA**.

The name may derive from the Indo-European **BHELENA**, meaning crazy plant, while in Proto-Germanic, the name **BIL**, meant vision, hallucination or magical power. A goddess named Bil, meaning exhaustion or moment, was an image in the moon or one of the moon's phases. She may have been the henbane fairy or goddess of the rainbow, as **BIL ROST** is the name of the rainbow bridge that leads to Asgard, and hence Heaven's bridge.

Hysocyamus is from the Greek **HYOSKYAMOS, HYS** meaning hog and **KYAMOS** meaning bean; thus hog bean, or swine's bean.

The ancient Sanskrit name Goat's Joy, was named after the animal's delight in feeding on the plant in small amounts.

Dioscorides suggested that pigs could eat the poisonous plant with impunity, and called the plant hycoscyhamos. He mentioned **DIOSKYAMOS** (bean of the gods, or Zeus' bean) as an outmoded name, possibly related to the plant's use in religious rituals. It was named **FABA JOVIS**, or Jupiter's Bean; and **HYPNOTIKON**, meaning sleep making.

Another common name, Insana referred to the drowsy and clumsy behaviour produced by the plant upon ingestion.

Niger is Latin for black, either referring to the plant's poisonous principals, or the ancient belief that if applied to any part of the human body, the part would turn black and rot.

The Greeks named it Apollinaris, in honor of the sun god, and used it in divination and as a narcotic. It was part of the incense that Pythia, of Delphi used to induce clairvoyance.

Henbane is an introduced annual or biennial with a heavy, unpleasant odour, that some call numbing. It is found on dry hillsides and wasteland. The leaves, when fresh, are even repulsive to mice and rats. When burned the leaves sparkle and smell like tobacco; and in some rural parts of England were smoked for relieving toothache. The dull, yellow seeds were placed on fires and inhaled for the same purpose.

In Medieval bathhouses, the seeds were roasted to create an erotic mood. Traditionally, in Afghanistan, the seeds were combined with Fly Agaric (*Amanita muscaria*), while in neighboring Pakistan they were smoked with tobacco or marijuana.

An archaeological dig south of Edinburgh of a 600 year-old hospital has revealed medicinal plant remnants in the ancient drainage system. Over 200 seed clumps have been found, one containing henbane (3 parts), hemlock and opium poppy (one part each). Checking the Augustinian monk's manuals revealed this mixture put the patient into a deep and pain free sleep for surgery.

The flowers are yellowish with purple veins. The plant in full flower smells like a mixture of fresh tobacco, black currants and musk, due in large part to content of tetra-methyl-putrescine. The Romans associated the plant with Jupiter.

Pliny recognized the psychogenic qualities of the plant and wrote.

“Henhane is of the nature of wine, and therefore offensive to the understanding, and troubles the head... used with great head and discretion. For this is certainly know, that, if one take of it in drink more than four leaves, it will put him beside himself. For mine owne part, I hold it to be a dangerous medicine, and not to be used but with great heed and discretion.”

It was considered most potent when gathered by a virgin standing on her right foot and picking the plant with her little finger. I’m not sure of this but I do know that one summer my herbal students picked the wild plant while in flower and going to seed.

Despite my warnings, one of the students processed the plant with bare hands and passed into a slumber for several hours. I am pretty sure she was not a virgin.

Baron Hammer-Purgstall believed “Bendj” to be the Nepenthe of Homer, a drug that was used to bring forgetfulness of sorrow or trouble.

The Roman historian, Josephus, infers the headdress of ancient Jewish high priests was modeled on henbane flowers.

An early contraceptive was made by mashing the seeds into paste with mare’s milk and tying the paste in a piece of wild bull’s skin.

The Old English Herbarium suggested plant juice for earache, swellings, toothache and painful breasts and genitals.

The ancient Gauls used henbane juice on their arrows and spearheads; while Egyptians put the seeds in their beer to make it more potent.

Cleopatra is said to have made use of the atropine in henbane for eye drops to make her pupils enlarged and more alluring. Egyptians smoked the leaves to relieve toothache.

Ancient German tribes used it as a tool of magic, and called it **BILSA,** or **PILSEN**. Pilsen chrut, and contemporary Bilsenkraut relate to its use in drinks of forgetfulness and erotic weather magic. For greater detail read *Symbolism and Mythology of Nature*, by Friedreich.

Beer made with henbane seed was very popular, as an aphrodisiac in Germany. Other herbs such as yarrow, labrador tea, and myrtle were used, and the beer consumed during the infamous drinking rounds was in honour of the god Aegir.

When the Bavarian Purity Law was passed in 1516, the use of henbane seeds was banned. Pilsen, or the drink of the devil, became a thing of the past, but lives on in the name of Pilsner beer.

The Celts named the plant **BELINUNTIA**, in honour of their sun god Bel. It is associated with the 11th Norse Rune, IS.

In the middle ages, it was used as an anesthetic like opium, mandrake, hemlock, aconite, or datura. In the form of a pomander (sleeping apple), or soporific sponge, it was used for narcotic inhalation. It was, in fact, an early "knock out drops". Witches and Monks of the era called it **INSANA**.

Flying ointments were said used by witches in the Middle Ages to fly to Sabbat on old pagan festival days. Henbane was part of these formulas, along with various nightshades, hemlock and monkshood. A German scholar Karl Kieswetter in 1902 made a sample of ointment from a traditional recipe.

After rubbing this into his skin, he fell asleep and dreamed of flying through the air. Professor Peuckert of Gottingen University had been studying folk tales of witches on broomsticks for over 40 years.

He discovered, in 1960, a flying ointment recipe in a book called *Magia Naturalis* by Johannes Porta, written in 1568, that included jimson weed, henbane and deadly nightshade. He substituted lard for baby fat (fair enough!) and decided to experiment on himself and a colleague. They applied the ointment to their wrists and forehead and within a few minutes were into a trancelike sleep that lasted for twenty hours. They each wrote down their experiences and later compared notes.

Both men reported sensations of flying through the air, and both had demonic visions. The good doctor reported landing on a hilltop and indulging in erotic rituals with naked women.

He believed that those who used the ointment reported similar experiences because the natural chemicals in the herbs stimulated areas of the brain responsible for "creating access to atavistic racial memories of pagan rites."

After eating too many Insana roots, one group of 19th century monks turned a pious convent into a madhouse when they insisted on chanting drinking songs instead of prayers.

Later, in England, Gerard and Culpepper both held Henbane in high regard. The latter herbalist wrote:

"The leaves cool inflammations of the eyes and any part of the body, and are good for the swelling of testicles, or women's breasts, or elsewhere, if they are boiled in wine, and either applied them selves, or the fomentation warm. The oil of the seed is good for deafness, noise and worms in the ears, being dropped there; the juice of the herb or roots act the same."

Anodyne necklaces were carved from the root and hung on the necks of epileptic children, or to suck when teething.

In North America, it escaped cultivation in 1670, and has been thriving ever since. Its introduction is said to be due to railroad builders who were in the habit of mixing the seeds with tobacco to strengthen the smoke.

The seeds are fatal to poultry and fish, and yet are mixed in feed for horses to fatten them.

The Eclectics, including Drs. Felter and King found it a very useful herb. In King's *American Dispensatory* is found the following:

"Hyoscyamus is a cerebro-spinal stimulant, or in the Eclectic meaning of the term, a cerebro-spinal sedative. It relieves pain and promotes sleep. Nervous irritation, without congestion, high fever, or disturbance of the circulation in the cerebrum is the keynote of its use.

In medicinal doses, it is anodyne, hypnotic, calmative and anti-spasmodic; allaying pain, soothing excitability, inducing sleep and arresting spasm. It does not produce constipation, like opium, but has a tendency to act as a laxative."

In 1910, Dr. Crippen used hyoscine to murder his wife, in a botanical whodunnit.

During the two World Wars, it was cultivated in small amounts in the United States.

In the late 1940s, annual production was around 38 metric tons. At one time it was extensively cultivated in Montana, thriving in elevations up to 7000 feet.

Today, the hand labor is too expensive, so it is cultivated on plantations in Turkey and India. The crude drug is the dried leaves, stems and flowering or fruiting tops. In annual varieties, the plant is harvested in flower.

In biennial forms, the non-flowering tops may be cut the first season, early the next spring and again during flowering. The root contains the highest concentration of alkaloids.

Its worst enemy is the Colorado potato beetle, which prefers this plant to all others; and a planting might even help the insects move away from your potatoes, another member of the nightshade family.

Sprays of the infused plant are effective against aphids on various fruit plants.

The related *H. physaloides* plant, including root, is used in Siberia as an inebriant and opium substitute.

Ancient Chinese used seeds and leaves in wine. The herb is known as **LANG TANG**.

MEDICINAL

CONSTITUENTS- seed- various alkaloids including atropine, hyoscine or scopolamine (highest in seeds), hyoscyamine (0.045-0.14%); tropine, atroscine, apogioscine, gossamide, and apoatropine; steroids including withanolides such as daturalactone-4, hyoscyamilactol, and 16alpha-acetoxyhyoscyamilactol; cannabisins D and G, as well as fatty oils mainly palmitin and olein.
The alkaline content of the leaf is from 0.35% to 1.4. The leaf also contains hyoscytricin, choline, calcium oxalate, potassium nitrate and fixed oils.
In young plant hyocosine dominates. Later, in the mature plant content is about 90% hyoscyamine, and scopolamine (1.2:1 ratio) with some atropine, and flavonoids including rutin; hyoscipirin, cuscohygrine, skimmianine, apohyoscine, alpha and beta belladonine, rutin, choline, mucilage, albumen, and potassium nitrate.
root- alkaloids above, as well as a several pyrrolidines including hygrine, as well as atropamine, tetramethyl-diamenobutane, and tropine.
hairy root culture- 12.5 mg/g alkaloids
flower- tetramethylputrescine

Henbane contains the alkaloids atropine, hyoscyamine and scopolamine, and is a central nervous system sedative for anxiety, depression, agitation and alcoholic delirium.

It is quite useful to allay irritability that leads to insomnia, in small doses. It is especially useful in mania, and the low, muttering delirium observed in some cases.

Because of its influence on the muscarinic receptors in the parasympathetic nervous system, henbane has been used for treating chorea and the tremor of Parkinson's disease.

It acts as a competitive antagonist with acetylcholine at nerve endings.

The dried leaves, flowers and seeds of commercial henbane are used for their alkaloids. They are usually administered in tranquilizers and sedatives for nervous infections, asthma, or whooping cough, and in tablet/dermal patch form for sea and air sickness. Until very recently, there was a great deal of variability in individual reaction to the patches. This appears to be mainly rectified.

Scopolamine or hyoscine is used prior to surgery to calm and sedate patients, while reducing saliva and incurring amnesia.

These same trans-dermal patches, containing hyoscine, are placed behind the ear of wind instrumentalists in orchestras to arrest salivation during a performance.

Hyoscyamine is the active ingredient in prescription drugs like Cytospaz and Urised, for cramping and spasms.

The whole plant is a powerful brain relaxant, anti-spasmodic on smooth muscle and sedative. It is vagolytic and useful for asthma as well as bronchial, gastric, intestinal, urinary and vascular spasms. Hyoscyamus is an ingredient in anti-asthma smoking mixtures.

It inhibits the release of acetylcholine as a neuro-transmitter, and produces a parasympathetic depressive or anticholinergic effect. The inhibition affects the muscarinic action of acetylcholine, but not the nicotine-like effects on nerve ganglia and motor end plates.

It exerts peripheral action on the autonomic nervous system; relieving nervous tremors of central nervous origin. It provides some relief in early stages of Parkinson's disease.

In moderate amounts it gently accelerates the circulation, producing gentle warmth on the surface and in the throat, causing sleep, headache, dilation of pupils.

The herb remains in several *South American Pharmacopoeia* for spasms of the urinary tract, and to alleviate the griping pain that is caused by purgatives.

Modern herbalists use henbane to help wean those coming off morphine, heroin, or cocaine habitual use.

It can be used as a hypnotic, where opium derivatives cannot be used, and is mildly laxative which opium is not. It is therefore the herb of choice in people with insomnia and children, where opium cannot be given.

Henbane lowers blood pressure through Ca++ antagonist activity. Khan et al, *Methods Find Exp Clin Pharmacol* 2008 30:4.

Henbane is a strong antidote to poisoning by mercury, at least in relieving the symptoms of heavy metal poisoning.

The leaves can be used as a poultice on painful rheumatism, gout, cancerous ulcers, and neuritis. A solid extract is used to produce suppositories that relieve hemorrhoid pain and swelling.

Whole plant extracts reveal activity against gram-positive bacteria.

The seeds are used in Traditional Chinese Medicine and known as **TIAN XIAN ZI**, meaning Fairy Lady Seeds, or sometimes **TIEN HSIEN TZU**. They are considered bitter and warm and used for their anti-spasmodic, sedative and analgesic properties. Uses include stomach cramps, heavy coughs, neuralgia and manic psychosis.

They are used in arthralgia due to wind, chronic diarrhea and dysentery and asthma with cough. Henbane seeds contain compounds that show moderate cytotoxic effect against human prostate cancer cell lines. Ma et al, *J Nat Prod* 65:12.

The roots are rich in alkaloids that diminish as the seeds mature.

HOMEOPATHY

Henbane (*Hyoscyamus*) is a remedy for the deeply disturbed nervous system. It is as if some diabolical force has taken possession of the brain, and prevented function.

It is the perfect picture of mania in a quarrelsome and obscene character. They are very talkative, and are want to removing clothing, and exhibitionism. They are jealous, fear being poisoned, and exhibit many of the traits of a weak and nervous agitation. They laugh at everything, exhibit low, muttering speech, and seem as if in a stupor.

There is great restlessness of both the nerves and muscles, with severe twitching, cramping of calves and toes, and spasms and convulsions.

The eyes have a glazed stare and unusual sheen, with protrusion, distortion and spasms of the eye muscles.

Dullness of vision, weakness and myopia, with marked pupil enlargement may be present.

There may be amaurosis, with flickering and dark spots in the field of vision, so that objects appear smaller, change position, or have blurred outlines. Objects appear in a scarlet light, or shining like gold.

There may be disturbance of hearing, with complete deafness; pains in the ear cartilage, and tearing pains, particularly in the evening.

Spasmodic tension and painful stiffness of the neck and shoulder muscles, along with tearing pains in the back and loins, and swelling of the ankle are present. There may be swelling and stiffness of the hands, with "pins and needles" types of pain.

Paralysis and coldness of the lower limbs, swelling of the feet with tearing pains in the soles, can occur.

Irregular heart beat with strong to weak pulse can be present.

It should be remembered for the symptom of grinding teeth at night.

Spasmodic coughs, particularly at night, are relieved by sitting up. There may be expectoration of green mucous with coughing, dryness of the throat, larynx and lungs.

Stomach pains, along with inflammation of the intestines are found, as well as retching, vomiting, and diarrhea.

The bladder may spasm, or paralysis of the bladder with frequent urging, and painful, scanty urination may be present.

In the male, there is temporary impotence with the need to expose oneself (flashers), or playing with genitals during fevers.

The female also has excited sexual desire, nymphomania, and inflamed conditions of the vaginal mucosa that is difficult to relieve. Menses may be too early and too heavy in some cases.

DOSE- Sixth to 200th potency. The mother tincture is made from the whole fresh plant in flower.

MATERIA POETICA

If you strut into my office
Naked as can be
Speaking lewdly to my staff
And grimacing at me
If you masturbate in public
And rant in jealousy
That would clue me into you
I'd know your remedy
It would be so nice and clear
If you could please arrange
To have a seizure with a shriek
Grind your teeth in your deep sleep
Lots of cursing when you speak
Show your fear of dogs and rats
Water running from the tap
You could become real manic
Dance wildly out of tune
Loudly incoherent
Pace around the room
These tips could really help me
To understand your role
It's shame and jealousy
That are central to your soul
And underneath betrayal
That cuts you to the quick
Oh to get your clothes back on
That will be the trick!

SYLVIA CHATROUX MD

PLANT OIL

A sun infused oil can be made from the whole fresh plant in flower or seed, using a 1: 5 ratio of plant to oil. Let stand for ten days, shaking daily, strain and preserve.

It is a useful oil in the treatment of scar tissue, and rheumatic pain, sciatica, earache and neuralgia. Be careful with preparation. A former student, who was well advised, handled the fresh plant material with bare hands, and fell into a four-hour slumber.

Oil of henbane combines well with belladonna, black nightshade, and the essential oils of lavender, peppermint, rosemary and thyme to make a tranquil balm.

The distilled oil could be used in rheumatic ointments if available. By destructive distillation the leaves yield very poisonous empyreumatic oil.

Henbane oil, particularly good for erotic massage, can be found in German pharmacies today.

SEED OIL

The seeds contain 0.093% alkaloids after crushing, including hyoscyamine. The fatty oil yield is about 25%, is an amber green colour, with a bland taste and very little odour.

It has a specific gravity of 0.9183; saponification of 191.72 and iodine number of 82.

HYDROSOL

Henbane water is good for them that have unnaturally…inwardly or outwardly of their body or head/the temples often times anointed therewith. Cloths wet in the water and laid upon the temples that causeth the person to his natural contentment. **BRUNSCHWIG**

FLOWER ESSENCES

Henbane flower essence is an aid in all stages of ego death, involved in real growth, often of a spiritual nature. This is frequently a Scorpio process, that reseeds the personality.

It can help adjust terminal patients to the transition into the next life. There may be euphoria. **PEGASUS**

Henbane is about making choices at the crossroads. When we made a flower essence with it, the flower itself, formed a triple crossroadpattern.

This geometric pattern links the flower to Hekate, crone goddess of thresholds, midwifery and magic, says Laurie Szott-Rogers in her book, Healing the Goddess Wound. www.selfhealdistributing.com

Hekate teaches us to manage the junctures in our lives, attuning to what we know and what we sense before deciding on a path.

The flower essence helps us understand that every path we take will have its own set of benefits and sacrifices. Taking a leap into the unknown is the only way to move forward. The sacrifice of leaving what is familiar is the cost of crossing the threshold. Trusting ourselves to handle what lies ahead allows us to enternew possibilities. Henbane is about making choices at the crossroads. **PRAIRIE DEVA**

PERSONALITY TRAITS

Let no one fill his belly, out of ignorance,
With Henbane, as men often do by fault or chance,
Or children who, from swaddling-clothes, headbands and need
To crawl unsurely on all fours but lately freed,
And walking upright, with no anxious nurse nearby,
Through witlessness chew on the baleful flower spray,
Since they are cutting incisor teeth along their jaws
Just then, which in their swollen gums sharp itchings cause.

NICANDER

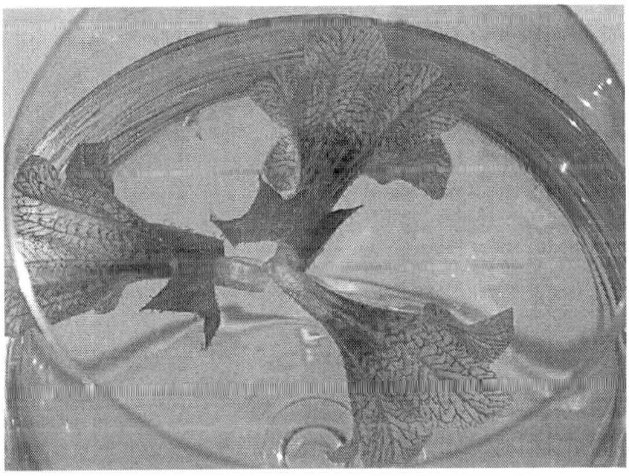
Preparing Henbane flower essence

Shameless, revealing and shocking are the threads that run right through [henbane], focused on sexuality. They may express this in sexually explicit ways, in obscenity and in pornography. For example, they can be embarrassingly frank when talking about personal things.

They use nakedness as a form of shocking, like the child who goes to the toilet and leaves the door open so they can be seen, or streakers, flashers, people who frequent nudist beaches or wear revealing clothes. They like being sexually shocking and offensive, in dress, in pictures, in drawings, in actions to disturb and gain attention.

A keynote is that their hand tends to gravitate to the genital area, inside their clothing in children...In extremes, a child will masturbate in front of visitors in order to shock and upset their parents. Extreme behavior is common. These people have a high sex drive and easy arousal and are extremely jealous...

There can be suspicion degenerating into deep mental states of paranoia with many delusions. They can pick at their clothes or play with their fingers, faces or lips. So when aspects of sexual shock, nakedness, masturbation, jealousy, muttering, bizarre tics, egotism, suspicion, sexual innuendo, pranks and deliberate anti-social behavior all occur together, this is the answer! **PETER CHAPPELL**

SPIRITUAL PROPERTIES

There are few plants which, at first sight, give such a mysterious, nay sinister impression as Henbane. The plant gives off an unpleasant musty-narcotic smell and feels sticky and oily. The flowers sit half-hidden in the foliage. They are of a dirty yellow colour with purple veins. Truly not a friendly looking flower!

The side branches reach out with an unusual but characteristic gesture like arms stretched upwards obliquely. An orderly double row of seed capsules extends along their length like vertebrae on a backbone. This impression of an animal's spine is enhanced by the curled-up head-like end of each branch. Only very few flowers are open at a time and they stand looking out like eyes in a forehead. With all its vegetative vigour it has not been able to maintain its pure plant nature. It is on the way to becoming part animal, and one must be really blind if one does not see it. **GROHMANN**

RECIPES

FLUID EXTRACT- Available as 1:1 ratios with total alkaloids of 0.045-0.055% and produced in a 20% alcohol from European firms. Dose-2-10 drops.

POWDERED HERB- 0.2 grams. In Britain the maximum dose is 100 mg and the daily dose no more than 300 mg. total. Dry extract 15-60 mg. Powdered leaves 2 to 10 grains. Up to 500 mg four times daily at upper end.

SEEDS- 0.6 to 1.2 grams.

TINCTURE- 3-10 drops. The fresh flowering tops make the best tincture at 1:2 and 50% alcohol. The dry plant should be prepared at 1:10 and 70%. For uterine cramps-5-10 drops twice daily.

FRESH LEAF JUICE- 2-4 ml.

INFUSION- 100-150 mg dried leaf.

JUICE EXRACT- The leaves are juiced, and then slowly evaporated to a thick consistency. It has a dark olive colour, with unpleasant odour, and a bitter, salty, nauseous taste.

HENBANE ALE- Take 40 grams of seed and bring to a boil in one litre of water. Remove from heat. Put 40 ounces of barley malt extract, 32 ounces honey and two litres of hot water in fermentation vessel. Add henbane, stir well and then add 24 litres of cool water. When in 68-76 F range, add yeast. Ferment. If desired, one ounce of sweet gale (*Myrica gale*) may be added to seeds in initial boil. **BUHNER**

NOTE: 1-2 pints of this ale are inebriating, while 1-2 litres are aphrodisiac. Henbane ale makes one thirstier the more one drinks.

CAUTION- Henbane is contraindicated in tachycardiac arrhythmias, prostatic adenoma, angle closure glaucoma, acute pulmonary edema, and mechanical stenoses in the area of the gastro-intestinal tract or enlarged colon.

Do not use in exhaustion, depression and feeble pulse.

Symptoms include impaired vision, heat build up due to reduced sweating, dry mouth, irregular heartbeat, enlarged pupils, delirium and severe constipation.

In overdose, begin gastric lavage, temperature-lowering measures with wet cloth (no antipyretics), oxygen, and diazepam for spasms, propranolol for tachycardia/arrhythmia.

In Traditional Chinese Medicine, licorice root is given to antidote henbane poisoning, but would only be of limited effect.

Do not combine with the following drugs: Amantadine (Symmetrel); tricyclic anti-depressants, anti-histamines, MAO inhibitors, narrow angle glaucoma drugs, Haldol, tranquilizers, Procanbid, and Quinidine.

In cases of severe poisoning, a slow intravenous administration of physostigmine is given until symptoms subside. This alkaloid is from the Calabar bean (*Physostigma venenosum*), originating in West Africa. If none handy, try large dose of lemon juice, or vinegar.

Or try an emetic of mustard, following by large amounts of warm water, strong tea or coffee with charcoal tablets. Apply heat and friction to extremities.

(LION'S MANE)
(POM-POM MUSHROOM)
(MONKEY HEAD)
(*H. erinaceus* [Bull.] Pers.**)**
(*H. erinaceum*)
(COMB TOOTH)
(BRANCHED HERICIUM)
(CORAL HEDGEHOG)
(BEAR'S HEAD TOOTH)
(*Hericium ramosum* f. caput-ursi [Fr.] D. Hall & D. E. Stuntz**)**
(*H. coralloides* [Scop] Pers.**)**
(*H. americanum* Ginns**)**
(*Hydnum erinaceum*)
CONIFER CORAL MUSHROOM
(*H. abietis* [Weir ex Hubert] K. A. Harrison**)**
PARTS USED- fruiting body, mycelium

Hericium means hedgehog from the Latin. Erinaceus is named after the European hedgehog, *Erinacius eruropeus*. Ramosum means branched. Coralloides means coral-like in reference to the distinct shape. Abietis is in reference to the genus Abies and growth on conifers. Lion's Mane is related to the fringed, hair-like appearance.

Comb Tooth must take the prize for most distinctive and beautiful fungi of the boreal forest. It is white, branched and covered with multitude of teeth that looks like ocean coral, or spongy icicles.

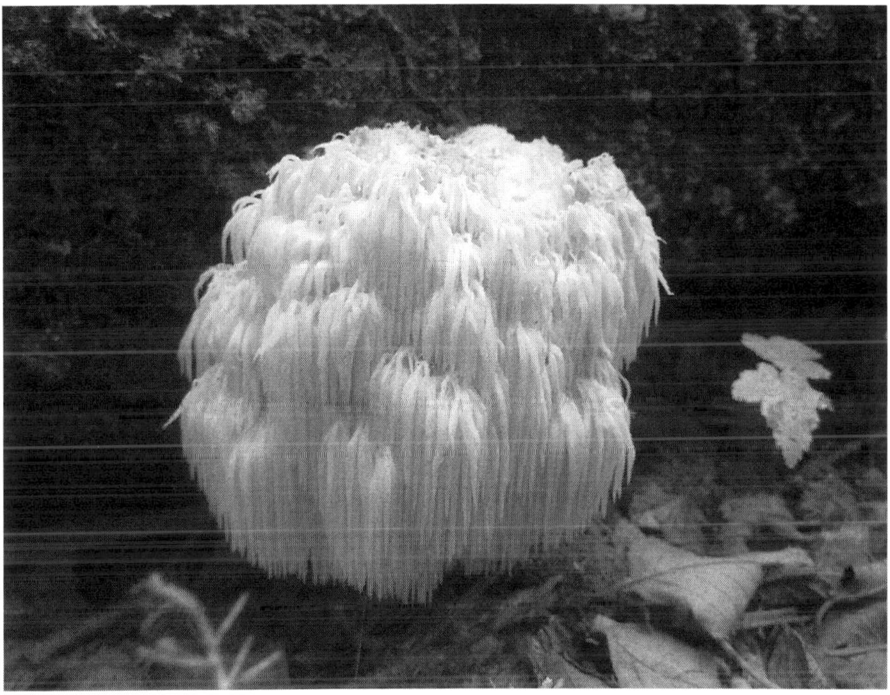

Lion's Mane (Courtesy of Gloria Arsenault)

It was one of three finalists in vote for Alberta's official mushroom, along with Oyster (*Pleurotus populinum*) and ultimate winner, Northern Redcap (*Leccinum boreale*).

It is edible and delicious sautéed in butter, especially when young, and is Laurie's absolute favourite. In fact, I often get to slip away to pick mushrooms on the off chance I will bring some of these Corals home.

Scientists have discovered an interesting compound, erinacine, found to be a kappa opioid receptor binding inhibitor. These are potent anti-convulsant compounds that can be neuro-protective in epilepsy, stroke, as well as brain and spinal cord injuries.

There is considerable taxonomic confusion between *H. americanum*, *H. coralloides* and *H. ramosum*. The latter species is believed by some authors, to be the former name of *H. coralloides*. The former mentioned is considered the new name for *H. coralloides*. Very confusing. On some forays, I have found the brain-like dense version on the same tree as the loose branched ones. I pick them all.

Here is my suggestion. The denser fruiting body may be considered *H. americanum*, the sparser *H. coralloides*, and drop *H. ramosum* altogether. The debate may go on for years. David Arora says the exact identity doesn't concern him, so I'll leave it at that.

Coral Hedgehog and Comb Tooth are found on hardwood species, especially poplar in Alberta. According to some authors, *H. coralloides* is found on both coniferous and hardwood trees.

Lion's Mane is used in Traditional Chinese Medicine for digestion and curing gastric ulcers. It has a tonic effect useful for treating neurasthenia and general debility.

Mycelium from various Hericium species extracted with hot water has been used in a sports drink called Houtou. This was a tonic used in the 11th Asia Sports Festival in 1990, and believed responsible for several victories.

I have not seen Lion's Mane on the prairies, but lots on Douglas Fir in British Columbia. Various Native tribes carried the dried powder in medicine bags as a styptic for cuts and wounds.

The Gitksan name is **KAEDATSOTS**, meaning bird hat, or hat of bird. Paul Stamets calls it a brain food that increases intellect and nourishes the nervous system. It is easy to inoculate conifer logs with plugs, sawdust or rope spawn, and grow your own.

In Japan, Lion's Mane is known as **YAMABUSHITAKE**.

Yamabushi means literally "those who sleep in the mountains" and relates to hermit monks from the Shugendo sect of ascetic Buddhism.

The mushroom is said to resemble the Suzukake, or ornamental garment, worn by these monks, and hence the name. In China, it is known as **SHISHIGASHIRA**, meaning "lion's head", or **HOUTOU**, meaning "baby monkey". Again, there is some controversy with some authors separating *H. erinaceus* and *H. erinaceum* into different species and other authors contend they are one and the same. It is found on oak from California north to Alaska.

Lion's Mane is delicious with a texture similar to seafood, and therefore grown commercially on a small scale. When served in French restaurants it is called Pom Pom du Blanc, due to the off white colour and shape resembling pom pom balls on the end of stocking caps or toques.

Research published in *Champignon* 2000 41:5 suggests the best medium for growing the fungi commercially is fine beech saw dust with 20% wheat bran.

Work by Poyedinok et al, *Int J Med Mush* 2005 7:3 found exposing mycelium to helium neon and argon laser irradiation increased growth, shortened the phases of mushroom development, produced more vigorous mycelium and increased fruit body yields from 36-51% in work on Lion's Mane, Oyster, and Shiitake.

Work by Suki Croan, *Forest Products Journal* 2004 54:2 found treating pine with extractive degrading fungi such as *Aureobasidium* spp., *Ceratocystis* spp., and *Ophiostoma spp.*, removed 70-99.9% of extractives. The treated wood chips were then used to cultivate *H. erinaceus*, as well as *Grifola frondosa* and various Oyster species.

Those wishing to grow the mushroom medicinally, should note that 26° Celsius is the optimal temperature, at 50-70% humidity, and that carbon dioxide levels can significantly increase growth.

Those interested in liquid culture will find a pH of 5, at 25° Celsius optimal. The best yields in fermenter cultivation use 20 grams inoculum per litre of nutrient solution. In two weeks, nearly 500 grams per litre can be realized. Contamination must be carefully controlled. Many substrates can be used for Hericium species production. For mycelium growth barley bran was best for *H. alpestre, H. lanciniatum* and *H. erinaceus, while H. americanum, H. coralloides* and *H. erinaceum* grew better on soybean powder. Ko et al, *Bioresour Technol* 2005 96:13.

Sunflower seed hulls have been used successfully with a 55-day cycle of growth from inoculation. Figlas et al, *Int J Med Mush* 2007 9.

Hericerin has been found to inhibit pollen growth. Kimura et al, *Agric Bio Chem* 1995 55.

MEDICINAL

CONSTITUENTS- *H. erinaceus*- beta-glucoxylan, glucoxylan, 31% protein, galacoxyloglucan protein, hericonene A and B (phenols), calciferol 240 IU/100 grams, ergosterol 381 mg/100 grams.

Polyhydroxysteroids include cerevisterol; six ergostane derivatives including; 3 beta, 5 alpha, 9 gamma-trihydoxy-ergosta-7, 22-dien-6-one; and the newly discovered 3 beta-glucopyranosul-5 alpha, 6 beta-di-hydroxyergosta-7, 22-diene, xylan, and glycoxylan. Cyathane derivatives are believed the nerve growth stimulators. Also contains the aromatic compounds erinacerins A and B.

Lion's Mane contains five polysaccharides and polypeptides that enhance the immune system, show significant inhibitory effect on sarcoma 180, and cancers of the stomach, esophagus and skin.

Ingestion of the mushroom in dried pill form has been found to extend the life of cancer patients.

Work by Okamoto et al, *Phytochemistry* 1994 34:5 showed activity against *Aspergillus niger*, and the yeast *Saccharomyces cervesiae*. They identified anti-microbial chlorinated orcinol deriviatives from the mycelium. Kawagishi et al, have a US patent (5,391,544) on cyathane derivatives of this mushroom, after finding it effective against aggressive HeLa cancer cell lines.

Y-A-2, reported by Mizuno in the 1999 *International Journal of Medicinal Mushrooms* is a newly discovered fatty acid component with pollen tube growth inhibiting activity, something shared with hericenone.

Mizuno has long been looking at this particular fungus, having identified Lion's Mane anti-tumour polysaccharides in *Biosci Biotech Biochem* 1992 56:2.

Both hericenone A and B appear to be directly active against cancer cells.

The mycelium is used in China to make pills for treating gastric and duodenal ulcers, as well as chronic gastritis.

It produces curative effect on both gastric and esophageal carcinoma. Work by Noor et al, *Int J Med Mush* 2008 10:4 found freeze-dried fruiting bodies provide cytoprotection against ethanol induced gastric ulcers in rats.

Lion's Mane is immune modulating, a nerve tonic and useful in chronic bronchitis. Wasser & Weiss *Critical Reviews in Immunology* 1999 19.

It is not directly chemotherapeutic, but works by stimulating the immune system, which in turn, helps control the growth of tumours. Son et al, *Int Immunpharmacol* 2006 6:8 found water extracts induce iNOS gene expression followed by NO production in macrophages via enhancement and activation of transcription factor NFkappaB.

Kim et al, *Phytother Res* 2009 May 13 found it increases human dendritic cells and re-inforces host innate immune system function.

Nagai et al, *J Nutr Biochem* 2006 17:8 identified di-linoleoyl-phosphatydl-ethanolamine as a compound that reduces ER stress and protects neuronal cells.

Hericenones C-H induce synthesis of nerve growth factor. This may be useful in the amelioration of Alzheimer's and other similar chronic nerve/brain related diseases. Kawagishi et al, *Tetrahedron Letters* 1991 32:35; 1994 35:10.

His work notes that the low molecular weight compounds pass through the blood brain barrier intact. Hericenones C-H, from fruiting bodies enhance nerve growth factor (NGF) production, useful for disorders of the peripheral nervous system.

Another class of cyathane derivatives from the mycelium, called erinacines A-I induce NGF production. Kawagishi et al, *Tetrahedron Letters* 1996 37.

The same author, in *Townsend Letter for Doctors and Patients* April 2004 makes a strong argument for the use of Lion's Mane for dementia. He suggests that erinacines are the most powerful inducers of NGF synthesis among all currently identified natural compounds.

A study of 100 patients in a rehab hospital in Japan, looked at the effect of five grams of Lion's Mane mushroom or placebo in their soup for six months. These patients were elderly and suffered from cerebro-vascular disease, degenerative orthopedic disease, Parkinson's disease, spino-cerebellar degeneration, diabetic neuropathy, spinal cord injury or disuse syndrome.

After six months, six out of seven dementia symptom patients taking the daily dose of mushroom demonstrated improvement in perceptual capacities and all seven had improvements in their Functional Independence Measure.

Lion's Mane may indeed be a potent inducer of brain tissue regeneration. Kasahara K et al, *Gunma Medical* Supp Issue 2001.

A follow up study was conducted with twenty-nine men and women aged fifty to eighty years, all suffering mild cognitive problems. Mori et al, *Biol Pharm Bull* 2008 31:9. In this double-blind (DB), placebo-controlled (PC) trial, significant improvement was shown in the mushroom group at eight, twelve and sixteen weeks. The dosage was just one gram of dried fruiting body three times a day in capsule form. All fourteen showed improvement after three months compared to placebo, but there was a decline four weeks after supplementation was discontinued.

The fruiting body may relieve depression, anxiety and insomnia in pre- and post-menopausal women. Mayumi et al, *Biomed Res* 2010 31:4. Thirty women aged 41.3± 5.6 years were given either cookies containing 0.5 grams of powdered fruiting body or no powder. Four cookies were eaten throughout the day. In this randomized, DB PC trial of four weeks, the participants filled out daily reports using four outcome measures. These were the Kupperman Menopausal Index (KMI), Centre for Epidemiologic Studies Depression scale (CES-D), Pittsburgh Sleep Quality Index and Indefinite Complaints Index (ICI). The latter was based on KMI but added items such as cognitive function, hair, skin, lower back pain, bladder and vaginal health measures.

No change was noted in sleep quality, but both CES-D and ICI mean scores were lower in the group taking enhanced cookies, compared to placebo. Anxiety and depression were lower, as well as comments associated with issues of frustration, palpitations, and increases in concentration and incentive.

Dr. Mizuno believes that these or similar compounds encourage the production of a protein called nerve growth factor, required by the brain for developing and maintaining important sensory neurons. Kolotushkina et al, *Fiziolog Zhurnal* 2003 49:1 found *in vitro* evidence of myelin generating effect on nerve and cerebellar glia cells.

Work by Moldavan et al, *Int J Med Mush* 2007 9:1 found extracts exerted neurotropic action and improved the myelination process in maturing fiber and did not exert a toxic effect, or cause nerve cell damage.

The compound 3-hydroxy-hericenone F, extracted and identified by Ueda et al, *Bioorg Med Chem* 16:21, shows protection against endoplasmic reticulum stress dependent Neuro2 cell death.

Water extracts of the fresh fruiting body given daily to rats with injured peri-neural nerves showed improvement in work by Wong et al, *Int J Med Mush* 2009 11:3.

A double-blind placebo-controlled trial of patients with cognitive difficulties found effective improvement with daily supplementation. Mori et al, *Phytother Res* 23:3.

Submerged mycelial extracts of *H. erinaceus* show anti-tumor activity on solid lymphoma. Krasnoolskaya et al, *Int J Med Mush* 2005 7:3.

Wang et al, *J Sci Food Ag* 2004 85:4 found methanol extracts of the fruiting body to possess hypoglycemic activity in a rat study.

Innovative work by Choi et al, *J Ethnopharm* 2005 100:1-2 cultured *H. erinaceus* on *Artemisia* species. When tested the methanol extract was found to inhibit proliferation of vascular smooth muscle cells. A methanol extract of the fungi showed no such activity, while an extract of *Artemisia iwayomogi* possessed strong inhibitory effects. The change of chemical components took place after addition of the Artemisia to the growth medium. The extract had strong protective effect on carbon tetrachloride hepatic damage in rats, with significant reduction in activity of GOT but not GPT and ALP.

Coral Hedgehog is used to cure gastric ulcers and has a tonic effect on digestion and the treatment of neurasthenia and general debility.

Early work by Harvey found activity against *Staphylococcus aureus*.

Erinacin E, from *H. coralloides/H. ramosum*, produced in a fermentation broth is a highly selective agonist of the kappa opiod receptor. It has an IC 50 of 0.8 μM, binding at the μ opiod receptor with an IC 50 of >200 mM.

These compounds may exhibit antinoceptive activity without the side effects associated with agonists like morphine. Saito et al, *Journal Antibiotics* 1998:15.

Herical, the precursor of erinacin E, was found cytotoxic and hemolytic in work by Anke et al, *Z Naturoforsch* 2002 57:3-4.

Total synthesis of this species has been reported by Watanabe & Nakada, *J Am Chem Soc* 2008 130:4.

The spent compost has been studied for industrial enzyme use, and found to contain alpha amylase (229 nkat/g), cellulase (759 nkat/g) and beta-glucosidase (767 nkat/g). Ko et al, *Folia Microbio* 2005 50:2. This suggests use in myco-remediation.

DOSE- Hericium extracts are standardized to 0.5% hericenones and 6% amyloban. Two capsules three to six times daily.

For gastric ulcers, decoct thirty grams of dried fruiting body in 500 ml of water for ten minutes. Divide in two doses and take twelve hours apart on empty stomach.

Dried powder can be put in 500-750 milligram vegetable or gelatin capsules. Or simply add to your daily smoothie or cooked cereal, soup or stew.

You can tincture the fresh fruiting body, and that is my favorite method. Use one part by weight to three parts of 60% alcohol. Dosage is from 5 to 10 ml twice daily.

For more medicinal mushroom information, see my book *The Fungal Pharmacy, The Complete Guide to Medicinal Mushrooms and Lichens of North America* by North Atlantic Books.

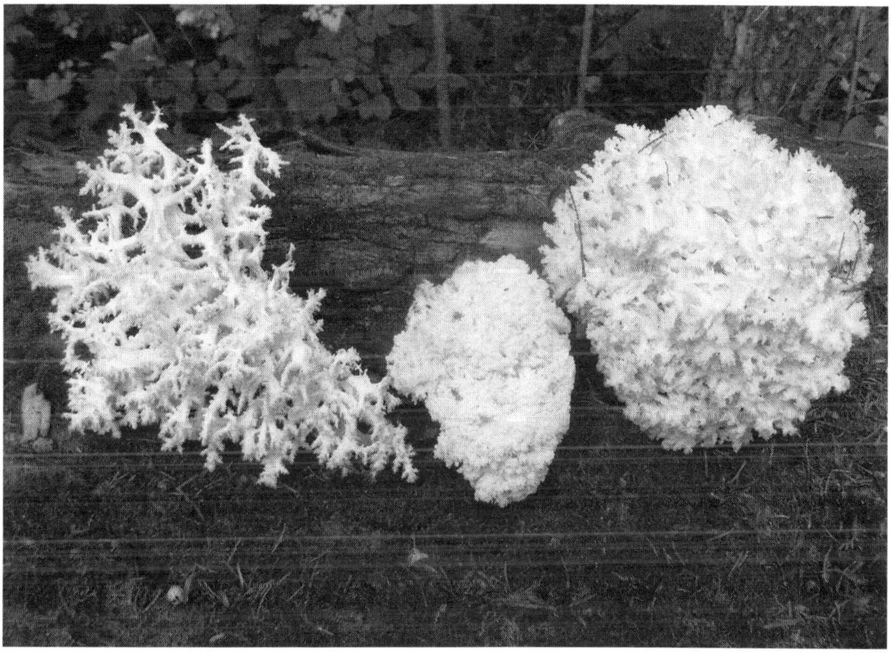

Three variations of *Hericium coralloides*

FIG MARIGOLD
CHANNA
KOUGOED
(*Sceletium tortuosum* [L.] N. E. Brown)
(*Mesembryanthemum tortuosum*)
ICE PLANT
(*M. crystallinum* L.)
(*Cryophytum crystallinum* [L.] N. E. Brown)

With pellucid studs the ice-flower gems
His rising foliage and his candied stems. **DARWIN**

Mesembryanthemum is from a Greek phrase roughly translating as flowers opening at midday.

This genus is originally from South Africa, but now planted as an annual ornamental all over the world.

In Morocco, *M. crystallinum* is used in soap making. Ancient Assyrians combined genus plants, known as **DILBAT**, with marijuana as a medicine for “suppressing the spirits”.

Despite their common name, they do not tolerate frost, but love the sun, opening only on sunny days. Ice plant refers to the ice-like shiny flecks on the leaves.

Several species including *M. crytallinum, M. expansum* and *M. tortuosum* are grown in prairie rock gardens, and drier soil.

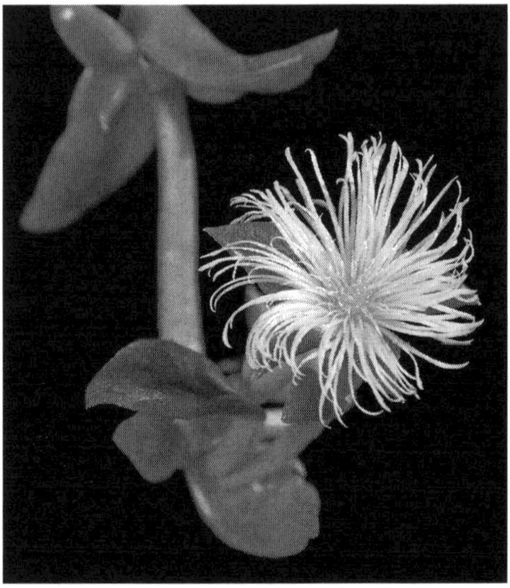

Kaugoed in bloom

The fermented plant is known as Kanna, or Channa, in its native country, and was used by the Hottentots as a narcotic, cocaine-like stimulant for more than two hundred years.

They chewed the root and kept it in their mouth for some time, until excited and intoxicated. When the Dutch arrived, they called it **KAUGOED**, meaning literally "chewable things".

Kolbe, an anthropologist of 260 years ago, wrote, "their animal spirits were awakened, their eyes sparkled and their faces manifested laughter and gaiety. Thousands of delightsome ideas appeared, and a pleasant jollity which enabled them to be amused by the simplest jests. By taking the substance to excess they lost consciousness and fell into a terrible delirium."

Laidler in 1928, noted that it was "chewed and retained in the mouth for awhile, when their spirits would rise, eyes brighten and faces take on a jovial air, and they would commence to dance."

Today, the root, leaves and bark of various ice plants are crushed, then chewed or smoked. Kaugoed (*S. tortuosum*) contains alkaloids with sedative activity. As little as five grams can create a state of stupor and lanquidity, and a prickly sensation on tongue. Higher doses can give a headache. It is used in South Africa as a narcotic to relieve pain, and as a party drug similar to use of *Cannabis sativa.*

MEDICINAL

The leaves of Fig Marigold are boiled to relieve fearful dreams associated with heart weakness. Investigation has found an ACE inhibitor in species. Duncan et al, *J Ethnopharm* 68 63-70.

It may be Africa's oldest natural mood enhancer and anti-depressant. It is stronger and works more quickly than St. John's wort.

Recent studies suggest it may be a phosphodiesterase inhibitor (PDE-4). These inhibitors augment intracellular secondary messenger signaling in brain cells and prevent the breakdown of key intracellular messenger, cyclic AMP involved in modulating multiple molecular processes involved in cognitive function, mood and inflammation.

Pharmaceutical PDE-4 inhibitors have undesired side effects, including nausea and vomiting. Harvey et al, *J Ethnopharm* 2011 137: 1124-1129.

One study, of an extract, Zembrin, on 36 healthy adults taking 8 mg or 25 mg for three months showed good tolerance. Nell H et al, *J Alter Complement Med* 201319(11).

Simon Chiu presented findings on Zembrin in twenty healthy adults in a DB, PC crossover clinical study. Twenty-five milligrams or placebo were given once a day for three weeks, then a three-week washout and a further switch with herb or placebo.

Compared to placebo, Zembrin at 25 mg per day selectively and significantly improved two key cognitive function domains, compromised by stress. Cognitive flexibility and executive function were improved, quality of sleep improved and the change in Hamilton Depression score also improved, albeit none of the 25 were depressed patients.

This suggests use for enhancing cognition during stress, improving cognitive decline in the elderly and treating neuro-degenerative disorders and mood-related conditions. Chiu et al, *Natural Bioactives International Conference* London, Ontario July 9-12, 2012.

A study of sixteen students, receiving 25 mg of Zembrin or placebo two hours prior to MRI scan revealed interesting results. During perceptual load task, amygdala reactivity to facial fear was significantly reduced compared to placebo. Emotion matching task showed activation of the midbrain, hypothalamus, amygdala and prefrontal cortex. There was a significant decrease in functional connectivity between amygdala and hypothalamus with Zembrin compared to placebo. This suggests reduction of anxiety-related effect. Terburg D et al, *Neuropsychopharmacology* 2014 38 2708-16.

The herb works by inhibiting serotonin (5-hydroxytryptamine reuptake transporters and selectively inhibiting phosphodiesterase-4 in CNS.

In 1914, Zwicky isolated the alkaloids mesembrine and mesembrenine. He dissolved 0.15 gram of mesembrine in hydrochloric acid, and heard buzzing in his ears, weakness of limbs and slight trembling. It also contains tortuosamine, all three interacting with the brain's dopamine and serotonin receptors. It elevates mood and decreases anxiety, stress and tension; and increases energy levels and concentration capabilities.

Mesembrenine demonstrates potent serotonin re-uptake inhibition, so interaction with various pharmaceuticals is a high probability. A US patent #8,552,051 has been awarded for mesembrenone, a key alkaloid for serotonin reuptake inhibition and PDE4, an enzyme that regulates the levels of cyclic AMP within the brain.

Shaman would mix the herb with ganja for that extra kick. It is often used as a tea to wean alcoholics off their favorite beverage.

It may cause a little nausea. Take on an empty stomach. Do not combine with *Rhodiola rosea*, as the combination makes you very tired.

Laboratory tests on frogs cause paralysis, and those on rabbits create convulsions. Don't give the herb to your pets!

Pinitol is a sugar alcohol, with a number of medicinal, commercial and industrial possibilities. When *M. crystallinum* is treated with 400 mM of NaCl, up to 70% of soluble carbohydrates in the plant are composed of pinitol. Control of light levels also affects pinitol production, making greenhouse propagation another source of this compound.

This plant, known also as *Cryophytum crystallinum,* is cultivated as a vegetable and salad. It was introduced into Germany for medicine around 1785 under the name Hottentot Fig.

After its introduction to the western states, it was used by cowboys as a sure cure for venereal diseases.

This tribe of the Kalahari Desert chewed or snuffed the dry root for psycho-activity. It contains mesembrine and oxalic acid.

Mesembrine and mesembrinine are analgesic and stimulate circulation, with the former also possessing cocaine-like properties. Some species contain N, N-DMT.

Mesembrine is a potent serotonin re-uptake inhibitor, similar in activity to Prozac. Preparations of *S. tortuosum* have been commercialized as anti-depressants to reduce anxiety. Frans Vermeulen and Linda Johnston report on symptoms associated with its use orally or smoked, in their giant four volume tome *Plants*.

"Walking was weird, there was something not-quite-right about my vision. It seemed like things were going by faster, or maybe slower, than I was walking past them.

The ground and walls seems to be moving past me either faster or slower than I was moving past them.

It seemed to take a very long time to get where I was going, but I never actually stopped on the way.

Some observed a ringing in ears, a caffeine-like buzz, with some euphoria."

The fruit of *M. acinaciforme* is used to treat pulmonary tuberculosis, while the root from *M. mahoni* is made into an intoxicating beer by the Bantu tribe, and into yeast for bread. The variety *M. stellatum,* or *Trichodiadema stellatum* is used for the same purpose.

Another related species, *M. edule* (*Carpobrotus edulis*) possesses sedative and psychotropic effect.

In Peru, one species is known as the Plant of the Maiden. Herbal amulets of the fleshy leaves are used by folk healers associated with the San Pedro cactus, as insurance "seguros" and in love magic.

COW ITCH
COWHAGE
VELVET BEAN
MUCUNA
(*Dolichos pruriens*)
(*Mucuna pruriens* [L.] DC.**)**
(*M. prurita*)
(*Stizolobium pruriens*)
PARTS USED- seed, pod hairs

Mucuna was a name used by Marggraf in the 1650s for a Brazilian species, from the Tupi word **MUCUMAN**. Cowhage or Cowage is derived from **KAWANCH** or **KOANCH**, two Hindustani words. The name has nothing to do with itchy cows.

Dolichos is from the Greek **DOLIKHOS**, meaning long or elongated.

Cowhage is a legume with white flowers and purple corolla, shaped like a butterfly. The flowers are dense and later form thick hairy pods that are brown and leathery in texture. It is a perennial in its native India, but may be cultivated here as an annual.

In 1688, the seeds were brought to London and exhibited as "itch powder".

The young pods are eaten as a vegetable in India and China, where they are known as **T'AO HUNG KING**.

The seeds, and pod hairs have a reputation in China as an aphrodisiac and anthelmintic.

For the latter, four or five hairs from the seedpod are taken with milk. The beans can be eaten like other legumes, or ground into flour and combined with other flours for bread. The seeds can be sprouted as well.

In the ancient Sanskrit and Ayurvedic traditions they are considered a potent aphrodisiac that promotes semen production and increases sexual vigour. In Sanskrit, the plant was known as **ATMAGUPTA**. It has been used to treat Parkinson's disease for over 4500 years, when the disease was called **KAMPA VATA**. James Parkinson re-described and renamed it in 1817.

In India, two ground seeds are taken in cow's milk as an aphrodisiac in the evening.

Mucuna is used in impotence, urinary disorders, leucorrhea, and spermatorrhea, prepared in a special powdered form.

The Bastar use seeds to increase semen production and cure nocturnal dreams, as well as diseases of the nervous system. The root was made into an ointment to treat elephantiasis.

In India, an extract of the root and seed were used in muscular atrophy and facial paralysis.

According to Leyel, the Pentaso believe the pods control the viscera, are a tonic to the marrow of the bones, and hence preserve life.

In Spain, the seeds are set in silver and worn to ward off the evil eye, and illness, known as **HABA**.

If eaten often enough, it will prevent hair from turning grey.

The seeds may be boiled in milk, decorticated, powdered and fried in butter. This is then made into a sweetmeat with twice its weight in sugar, and given to those suffering paralysis.

In Mexico, the seed is also used for its potent aphrodisiac activity, and in Brazil as a sexual and nerve tonic. The crushed seeds are taken with sugarcane juice in Trinidad for intestinal worms. In Guatemala it is known as Nescafe, due to its use roasted and ground as a coffee substitute. In Guatemala? Don't they have good coffee beans?

In Nigeria, the hairs are mixed with honey for intestinal worms. Salve of the hair and fat is used in Ethiopia for rheumatism.

The plant is used in veterinary medicine for urinary complaints, elephantiasis, anthrax, tympanitis, and lumbar fracture.

In parts of Africa, the spicules, or itching hairs, are used as part of NSU poison.

In Southeast Asia the root and hull decoctions are taken as a diuretic and to alleviate sinus and nasal inflammation.

The leaves are dried and can be smoked.

Combined with harmaline source plants, it stimulates the CNS and colorful geometric patterns that later spiral around the smoker.

Richard Schultes and Albert Hoffman, in *Plants of the Gods*, wrote, "the total indole alkylamine content was studied from the point of view of its hallucinogenic activity.

It was found that marked behavioral changes occurred which could be equated with hallucinogenic activity".

The plant and seeds contain the psychoactive DMT and 5-MeO-DMT. See Reed Canary Grass. A report out of Mozambique found 203 cases of acute toxic psychosis associated with eating the seeds as an alternate food source.

Headaches, palpitations, hallucinations and paranoid delusions were present, and all recovered within two weeks. Infante et al, *Lancet* 1990 336 1129.

MEDICINAL

CONSTITUENTS- *Mucuna pruriens* seed- L-dopa (3,4 dihydroxyphenylalanine, amines such as 5-hydroxy-tryptamine (serotonin), N,N-dimethyl-tryptamine, bufotenine, bufotenidine, a 5-oxindole-3-alkylamine derivative, DMT, DMT-N-oxide, N,N-DMT, 5-MeO-DMT, two beta carbolines, various amino acids, globulins, albumins and the alkaloids mucunadine, mucunine, prurienine, prurieninine, prurienidine, mucunadine, mucuadinine; as well as mucuanain, a proteolytic enzyme, cytisine, tyrosine and nicotine.
Various fatty acids as well as lauric acid, lecithin, D-galactose and D-mannose also present in bean.
Pods- serotonin, indole-3-alkylamines-N, N-dimethyltryptamine, bufotenine.
Root- beta sitosterol, stigmasterol, beta amyrin acetate, ursolic acid, betulinic acid
Leaf- tryptamines, 6-methoxyharman
Seedpod hairs- aproteine andmucunaine.

Cowhage, or Velvet Bean is both rubefacient and anthelmintic. The indole bases are reported to be spasmolytic and to depress respiration and blood pressure; as well as reduce blood sugar and cholesterol serum levels.

Work by Akhtar et al, *Journal Pak Med Assoc* 1990 40 and Grover et al, *J Ethnopharm* 2001 76 found hypoglycemic effects in alloxan and streptoxotocin diabetic mice, respectively. This effect was partially dependent on stimulation of functional insulin-producing beta cells.

Rathi et al, *Phytother Res* 2002 16 showed diabetic rats treated with the bean for four months exhibited a 51% drop in plasma glucose levels. Work by Donati in same journal 19:12 identified d-chiro-inositol 2 galacto derivatives as possessing anti-diabetic activity.

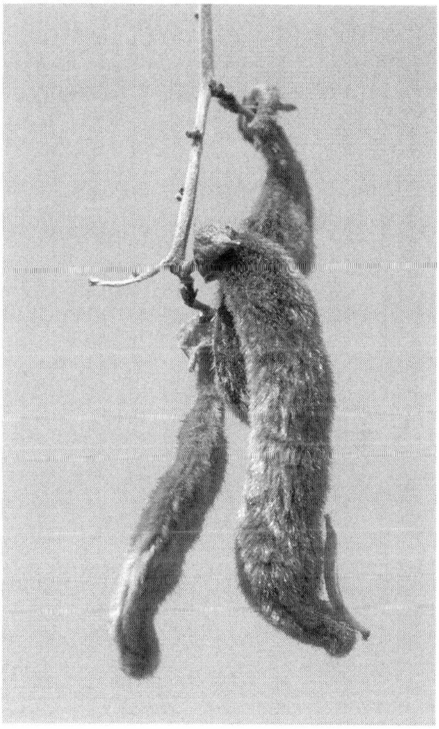

Velvet Bean
(*Mucuna pruriens*)

Medicarpin and parvisoflavone are potent alpha glucosidase inhibitors (two fold less active than acarbose). Dendup T et al, *Planta Medica* 2014 80(7): 604-8.

The beans are high in trypsin and chymotrypsin that aid in digestive processes.

As well as traditional usage as an aphrodisiac, the plant is used to allay depression, enhance alertness and improve coordination. One study in India looked at 25 patients with depressive illness. A dose of 3 grams of seed showed increased levels of dopamine, serotonin and other catecholamines in the brain that induce mood elevation.

Several clinical trials show increased sexual and androgenic activity.

The seeds are taken orally by men to promote fertility and as an aphrodisiac to increase seminal fluid and vigor. Two seeds are traditionally powdered and taken with a cup of cow's milk.

Hot water extracts are taken as a nervine and to promote delayed menstruation.

A clinical trial of 133 subjects aged 18-46 presented cases of improper erection, night emissions, premature ejaculation, spermatorrhea, functional impotence and/or oligospermia, with 71% claiming aid from the herbal extract.

Another study involved an herbal combination including *Mucuna pruriens*, *Tribulus terrestris* and licorice root, on 56 subjects with sexual dysfunction for four weeks.

Improvement in erection, duration of coitus and ejaculation as well as post coital satisfaction was noted.

Work by Ahmad et al, *Fert Steril* 2008 90:3 found 300 mg doses given to 60 fertile and 60 infertile males increased sperm count and motility in the latter group significantly.

In a study of 180 infertile men and 50 healthy men as control, the herb was found to improve the semen quality. It reactivated the enzymatic activity of metabolic pathways and energy metabolism, as well as rejuvenated the harmonic balance of male reproductive hormones in infertile men. Gupta A et al, *J Pharm Biomed Anal* 2011 55:5.

Other studies indicate hypo-prolactinaemic, hypoglycemic, spermatogenic, anabolic, and anti-inflammatory activity.

Vaidya et al, *Neurology* 1978 26:4 found 15 grams of seed powder as effective as 0.5 grams of L-dopa.

L-dopa, converted to dopamine stimulates the release of growth hormone by pituitary gland. It is also an effective inhibitor of prolactin, and increased levels of this compound are associated with erection dysfunction in males.

Mucuna seed, according to some sources, contains 5-methyl N, N-dimethyl-tryptamine, or serotonin; while other sources say 3,4 dihydroxy-phenylalanine. DMT is, in concentrated form, a hallucinogen that increases perceptional distortions.

Mucuna contains natural dopamine that shows a protective effect in Parkinson's disease. In one study, the dopamine content was separated and the bean still showed effect on the disease, suggesting that more than dopamine agents are at work. Hussain et al, *Phyto Res* 1997 11:6. It may well be that unidentified compounds enhance L-dopa efficacy, or other anti-Parkinsonian compounds are present.

L-dopa is the naturally occurring form of the amino acid 3,4 dihydroxy-phenylalanine, a precursor to norepinephrine and epinephrine, and melanin, a pigment in the hair, skin and substantia nigra of the brain. It is classified as a natural product in Sweden.

A randomized, double blind controlled trial with eight Parkinson's disease patients found 30 gram preparations led to "considerably faster onset of effect" in comparison to standard L-dopa/carbidopa pharmaceuticals, concluding that "this natural source of L-dopa might possess advantages over conventional L-dopa preparations in the long term management of PD". Katzenschlager et al, *J Neurol Neurosurg Psychiatry* 2004 75:12 1672-77.

Studies suggest mucuna endocarp powder acts on a novel mechanism that is different than l-dopa, and without causing dyskinesia. Lieu CA et al, *Evid Based Compl Altern Med* 2002 September 10.

L-dopa promotes sleep and has been found to advance the circadian rhythm of sleep. Lack of dopamine is related to restless leg syndrome and may help this sleep disorder as well.

Seed sprouts inhibit alpha amylase and alpha glucosidase and are optimal after four days germinating in dark. Optimal levels of L-dopa are found after one day of sprouting. Randhir et al, *Bioresourc Tech* 2009 100:19.

Mucuna reduced paraquat induced Parkinsonian mouse neurotoxicity. Yadav SK et al, *Neurochem* 2013 62:8.

The seed is a CNS stimulant in low doses, and depressant at higher doses.

The bean contains bufotenine, a cholinesterase inhibitor; mucunain, an anthelmintic; and serotonin that relaxes muscles, reduces cholinesterase and intestinal gas, and acts as a clotting agent.

5-Methoxy-DMT is the most effective hallucinogenic after LSD-25, and is clearly stronger than T-hydroxy-DMT and DMT. Fabing and Hawkins, *Science* 1956 123 886-7.

Velvet Bean is increasingly found in various weight loss, libido, brain/ memory, anti-ageing and body building formulas.

Persons with androgenic excess syndrome should avoid velvet bean.

Hirsutism, or polycystic ovary syndrome is a prevalent cause/effect of elevated androgen. One third of PCOS women have elevated androgens and about 10% type 2 diabetes.

In males, cystic acne and male pattern baldness are related to hyper-androgenism. Internationally, the incidence of androgen excess is an estimated 8% of population!

The cotyledon powder shows anti-parkinson's activity superior to synthetic levodopa. Tharakan et al, *Phytother Res* July 11, 2007. This may be due to GnRH agonist activity according to the authors.

A 2004 rat study found the cotyledon powder significantly restored endogenous levodopa, dopamine, norepinephrine and serotonin content in the *substantia nigra*.

Indole alkylamines showed hallucinogenic activity in work by Bhattacharya et al, *Ind J Physio Allied Sciences* 1971 25:2.

Cotyledon powder has been found to restore endogenous levodopa, dopamine, norepinephrine and serotonin levels in work by Manyam et al, *Phyto Res* 18:9.

In a human study, the bean powder was given to 60 patients with significant reduction of parkinson's symptoms.

The beans are placed on hot charcoal and the fumes inhaled for persistent cough.

Ethanol extracts of the dried trichomes show analgesic and anti-inflammatory activity.

The dried root powder is taken with honey as a blood purifier, diuretic and to help dissolve kidney stones.

Velvet bean also prolongs the time needed for blood to clot, suggesting a blood-thinning agent. The pod hairs are extremely irritating to the skin, and must be handled with care.

HOMEOPATHY

Dolichos (Cowhage) is a right-sided medicine with pronounced liver and skin symptoms. There is a general intense itching without eruptions, as well as senile pruritis and hemorrhoid diathesis.

Pain in the throat, made worse by swallowing that feels as if a splinter were imbedded. Pain from the gums may prevent sleep.

Colic may occur from dampness and getting wet feet. Constipation with intense itching, a bloated abdomen, white stools, swollen liver, and burning hemorrhoids are all possible indications for its use.

The intense skin itching is worse across the shoulders, and about the knees, elbows and hairy parts. Herpes zoster may be relieved.

The itching is made worse by scratching, is worse at night and on the right side of the body.

Stunned, as if received a blow to head. Taste of blood in mouth and cough.

DOSE- Sixth potency. For hemorrhoids, use drop doses of the mother tincture. The mother tincture is prepared from the dried hairs from the pods of the plant *Dolichos pruriens*. A self-experiment was conducted by Jeanes at 2c dilution in 1838. MacFarlan did proving with same potency in 1890s. May be trialed at 6X for hirsutism and polycystic ovary syndrome.

RECIPES

POWDER- Up to 5 grams daily.

CAUTION- The bean is androgenic and should be avoided in those with PCOS.

LESSER PERIWINKLE
COMMON PERIWINKLE
(*Vinca minor* L.)
HERBACEOUS PERIWINKLE
(*V. herbacea* L.)
PARTS USED-whole plant above ground

"Through primrose tufts in that sweet bower, the fair periwinkle trailed its wreaths." **WORDSWORTH**

Vinca is from the Latin **VINICO** meaning "to bind", and refers to the strong, sprawling stems that bind and stunt competing plants. Vinca is the past tense of the verb **VINCERE**, meaning to conquer, overcome or overpower. **PER** means through; and **PERVINCA** was the name given the plant by Pliny the Elder. It may derive from the Russian **PERVI** meaning first, in reference to early spring.

So the name, either to bind closely, or to overcome, is still up in the air, scholastically speaking.

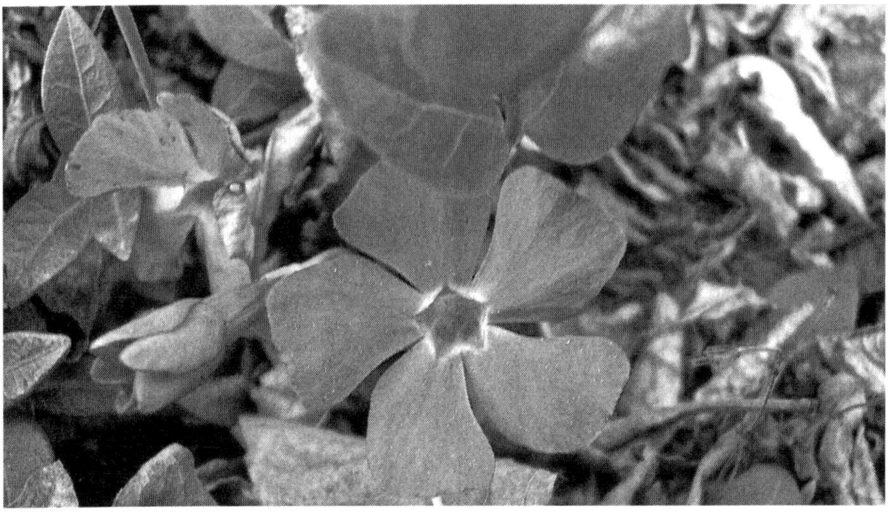

Periwinkle in flower

An early translation of Book of Secrets attributes Albertus Magnus to the following statement.

"Periwinkle when it is beate to a poudr with worms of ye earth wrapped about it and with an herbe called houselyke, induces love between a man and his wife if it be used in their meals."

Periwinkle was, at one time, believed to help those suffering nightmares.

About 22 years ago, my wife, Laurie, and I bought a home in the southern burbs of Edmonton. We moved in October, with the ground covered in white snow.

The following spring, as the snow was melting, I noticed our neighbor's ground cover with shiny dark green leaves moving into our yard.

And it soon blossomed with beautiful sky-blue flowers. The plant is an evergreen perennial that flowers, but rarely ripens to seed on the prairies.

When my neighbor told me he thought it was periwinkle, I didn't really believe him. But I scurried back to my herbal books. Sure enough!

It was introduced to our region by early Ukrainian settlers; and is known as Barvenok.

In the rhyme for new bride's apparel, the something blue may be blue periwinkle, for in parts of England, it is worn in the garter for fertility.

Periwinkle is often planted in newly weds yards to ensure a lucky and happy marriage. Other magical properties have been associated with periwinkle. It was believed that if a husband and wife ate the leaves together, it would bind them more closely. It has come to symbolize pleasant recollections, and associated with birth date of March 28.

European peasants used the herb to both dry up over-abundant milk production, or to dry off in late stages of pregnancy. It is also used for chronic diarrhea, and to arrest bleeding wounds, and internal hemorrhage.

According to Grieve, it as a familiar flower in the days of Chaucer, who called it "fresh Pervinke rich of hue". Bacon says that bands of periwinkle stem tied around a limb prevent or relieve cramp.

An older name was "Sorcerer's Violet", as it was believed to exorcise evil. In parts of England, garlands of periwinkle were placed on prisoner's heads before execution. Vinca pervinca became periwinke. Another name Saint Candida's Eyes, from western Dorset, refers to a medieval healer.

In France it is sometimes referred to as "the violet of witches".

In Italy, it was known as **FIORE DI MORTE**, or flower of death, for its use as decoration on the funeral pyres of deceased children.

Herbarium, written by the 2nd century AD writer Apuleius, described vinca minor virtues "against the devil sickness and demonical possessions and against snakes and wild beasts". For snakebites, it was steeped in vinegar, and taken internally to neutralize the venom.

Vinca minor is a great protector, and is gathered when the moon is 9 nights old, according to tradition. That is, nine lunar months into the new year.

The Italians call it **CENTOCCHIO** or hundred eyes, to the Germans it is the "Flower of Immortality" and to the French it is an emblem of friendship.

The Cree of Alberta named the introduced plant, **KA PAPAMIKIHK WAPIKWANE**, a trailing evergreen flower.

An old recipe for inducing love between a man and wife was a mixture of periwinkle, houseleek, and earthworm, somehow disguised in a meal. Children enjoy the small fairy-like paintbrush left over after all the petals have been removed.

Culpepper said it was good for bleeding of the mouth and nose when chewed; and useful in hysteria and fits. "It is good in nervous disorders, the young tops made into a conserve is good for the nightmare."

In Somerset, decoctions of the stem were taking to prevent cramps.

Medieval herbalists prescribed *Vinca minor* for headaches, vertigo and memory loss.

For whitlows, or other skin growths associated with poor circulation, a bath decoction is used to bathe the affected area with excellent results. Another name, Cutfinger, refers to its healing properties of skin.

The root is used in sub-Saharan Africa to treat hypertension, while in Norway the fresh leaf is given for internal hemorrhage, especially after injury.

Herbaceous periwinkle looks similar but is only of medium hardiness.

Vinca major, a variegated perennial, is sold on the prairie regions as an annual that flowers the first year from seed. It is not very hardy, but in milder climates is used as a perennial ground cover.

MEDICINAL

CONSTITUENTS- *V. minor-* over 70 carboline, dimeric imidazolidino-carbazole and quaternary alkaloids (0.58-0.85%) including vincamine (200-17,500 ppm), vincarubine,vicarine, vincine, vincaminorine, vincaminoreine, apovincamine, and vincadifformine; 30 indole alkaoids of the eburnan type; 1-norvincorine; 4-methyl-raucubainum chloride, 4-methylstrictaminium choride, and 4-methyl-akummicinium chloride; akumnicine, akuammine, akuammine N-oxide, ervine, isomajdine, majdinine, reserpinine, resperine, robinin; and various uncharacterized alkaloids including minoveinceine, vincareine, vincoridine, vinerine, tombozine, vincamajine, vincorine, vinomine, and vinoxine.

V. herbacea- vincanine, majdine, isomajdine, norfluoro-curarine, hervin, akuammicine, dl-vincadiffornnine, akuammine, carapanaubine, ervine, vincaherbinine, herboksine, isomajdine, isoresperpinine, majdine, 11-methoxy-vincadifformine, vincarine (0.064% dry weight), herbadine (0.081%), herbamine (0.077%), reserpinine, skimmianine, tabersonine, venalstonine, vincamajine, N-oxide, vincalines,and tabersonine.

Lesser Periwinkle (*V. minor*) has long been used in herbal medicine for its purgative effect. The fresh leaves are an excellent gentle laxative for young children, and for chronic constipation in the elderly, but used with care. It can also be used for the milk crust on scalp common to young children.

The fresh flowers can be made into a laxative syrup, by simmering them in honey or maple/birch syrup for about ten minutes. James Duke reports that the flowers "are said to be poisonous", but I have eaten them with no ill effect.

The leaves possess stomachic and bitter properties, useful in chronic stomach belching, intestinal inflammation and flatulence; combining well with *Agrimony.*

It possesses astringent and tonic properties useful in uterine hemorrhage; in between period bleeding and excessive menstrual flow during menopause.

Lesser Periwinkle will also help decrease the flow and quantity of breast milk, when applied as a heated poultice externally.

It clears mucous from the lungs, and intestinal tract; and as an astringent gargle will relieve sore throats, tonsillitis, canker sores, and the irritating crust formation with the nasal septa.

For bleeding hemorrhoids and internal hemorrhage it may be taken internally, as well as applied externally, or taken as a retention enema.

Michael Moore used the closely related *Vinca major* for migraine headaches that occur after adrenaline stress from circumstance or rebound reaction of low blood sugar from skipping meals. He suggests it be used for short-term acute use, as this is a complex alkaloid plant.

Chewing the fresh leaf will give quick relief to toothache.

It combines well with *Ginkgo biloba* to stimulate vascular and cerebral circulation.

It is good for cerebral insufficiency, "yin" migraines, for impaired memory and cognitive function, behaviour disorders, irritability, restlessness, and speech disorders.

It is very useful for poor circulation to peripheral areas of the body- hands, feet and brain, in cases associated with diabetes and atherosclerosis.

Water extracts of leaves and ethanol extracts of flowers exhibit strong anti-tumor activity. Yildirim AB et al, *Asian Pac J Trop Med* 2013 6:8 616-24.

Vincamine was extracted from the leaves industrially in 1955, and has been used for treating cerebrovascular problems since 1959. It is recommended for tinnitus and Meniere's disease. For this purpose vincamine is used 20 mg three times daily.

Vincamine is a muscle relaxant.

One team of researchers summarized their findings as follows: "The trends discovered with ECG monitoring show that vincamine undoubtedly improves the diffuse changes in electrical activity in the brain.

This improvement in the whole cerebral vascular system is all the more interesting if one considers how difficult it is to interpret changes in human cerebral metabolism."

Vincamine has been used for insufficient flow of blood to the brain, difficulty sleeping, mood changes, depression, hearing problems and high blood pressure.

Vinpocetine is produced by transforming the chemical structure of vincamine. It is a cis(3S,16S)-derivative of vincamine with anti-anoxic, anti-ischemic and neuro-protective properties.

Vinpocetine has been widely studied for the treatment of tinnitus. Konope et al, *Otol Pol* 1997 51; Ordogh et al, *Ther Hungarica* 1978 26; Ribari et al, *Arzn Forsch* 1976 10.

Vincopetine prevents the accumulation of sodium in brain cells, lowering their overall charge and preventing tissue destruction reactions of sodium and oxygen when circulation is restored after stroke. It also possesses calcium channel blocking activity and phosphodiesterase inhibition.

Phosphodiesterase is the enzyme responsible for breaking down ATP, or adenosine triphosphate, which is the primary energy of all cells. The inhibition is specific to the brain, resulting in localized increase in energy to neurons.

Vinpocetine is not only a cerebral vasodilator, but selectively enhances circulation and oxygen use with increasing systemic circulation.

It also inhibits platelet aggregation and decreases deformity of red blood cells. Kuzuya, *Therapia Hungarica* 1985 33.

Vinpocetine enhances both glycolytic and oxidative reactions of glucose breakdown in brain. Vamosi et al, *Arzn Forsch* 1976 28.

It does all this without significantly affecting systemic blood pressure and without serious side effects.

The herb can be of use in treating brain trauma, and disorders of blood flow to the retina.

Clinical studies have shown vinpocetine helps maintain healthy microcirculation to the eyes and inner ear. One study of patients with mild burn trauma to eyes showed enhanced healing, due to increased blood flow to damaged tissue.

It is approved for use in 47 countries, and has been in clinical practice since 1978. The Hungarian company Gedeon Richter markets vinpocetine under the drug name Cavinton for the treatment of various cerebral insufficiency conditions. In one study with Cavinton on cerebral glucose metabolism in chronic stroke patients, the drug shows significant improvement in transport of glucose to the brain tissue damaged by stroke.

Periwinkle can be used to dry up an overly abundant milk flow in animals, or to dry off when in later stages of pregnancy.

The root is hypotensive, and used for high blood pressure. It acts on the central nervous system as a sedative. It is adrenolytic and lowers the peripheral resistance.

Lesser Periwinkle show not be confused with *Vinca rosea* from Madagascar, from which alkaloids have been isolated and used successfully in various childhood leukemia.

However, Sturdikova et al, *Pharmazie* 1986 41:4 have shown three alkaloids from *Vinca minor* to possess cytotoxic and anti-tumour activity. They had considerable inhibitory effect on leukemia P388 cells, with vincadifformine the most active, stopping cell proliferation *in vitro* at 50 mcg/litre concentration even after twelve hours. The activity was greater than vinblastine, derived from unrelated Madagascar Periwinkle.

The plant is cytotoxic to HT29, Caco2 and T47D cancer cell lines. Khanavi et al, *Pharm Biol* 2010 48:1.

The alkaloid content is highest during flowering and fruiting; and should be collected at this time. Water extracts of the leaves show activity against gram-positive bacteria.

In France, the extract vincamine is prescribed at 40-60 mg/day for a variety of cerebral senility problems. It is contra-indicated in cerebral tumours with intracranial hypertension, and in pregnant women.

One study of the elderly, involved 30 mg for 12 weeks for primary degenerative and vascular dementia on 152 patients aged fifty to eighty-five. Therapeutic efficacy was shown in this study.

Dr. Weiss reports very good results with *V. minor* in cases of Meniere's disease and tinnitus. In one study of treating hearing loss after acoustic trauma, improved hearing was found in 79% of patients, and improved tinnitus in 66%.

Robinin, a flavonol 0-glycoside, is an HIV-I protease inhibitor.

Vinpocetine has been the subject of over 300 studies published in medical journals. Vinpocetine is a vincamine derivative, and a synthetic ethyl ester of apovincamine. It is also known as Intelectol, Calan and simply Vinpocetine as a brand name.

Vinpocetine has been shown to increase production of the neurotransmitters norepinephrine and dopamine, and increase the release of serotonin. It is considered a pro-acetylcholine as it increases concentration and may help alleviate depression via the increase in serotonin levels.

It inhibits acetylcholine release provoked by glutamine (MSG) and other neuro-excitory amino acids.

More importantly, it is a powerful vasodilator that relaxes the smooth muscles of the vessels leading to the brain, making more oxygen and glucose available to the brain. Combining with a source of rutin, such as buckwheat or violet leaf is even better.

It inhibits cyclic GMP phosphodiesterase, and speculated to enhance cyclic GMP levels in vascular smooth muscle. This is probably the route of increasing blood flow to the brain.

It inhibits platelet aggregation and increases the deformability of red blood cells of erythrocytes, reducing blood viscosity and enhancing mircro-circulation. Schmid-Schonbein et al, *Drug Dev Res* 1988 14.

Vinpocetine may be useful in alleviating migraine headaches, including those associated with PMS.

Vinpocetine may help in the prevention of gastric ulcers, inhibiting the development of lesions. Nosalova et al, *Arzn Forsh* 1993 43.

Interesting work by Miyata et al at the Taisho Pharmaceutical Company in Japan found blood levels of alkaline phosphatase and bone osteocalcin decreased after ingesting vinpocetine. The study looked at kidney dialysis patients, with administration of 15 mg daily for 3-12 months leading to complete elimination of calcinosis in all eight patients.

Some herbalists find it useful in treating retinitis, combining well with pulsatilla. It may be tried in retinopathy, which is a more chronic condition characterized by congested blood flow, combining with bilberry fruit. Work by Kaham et al, *Arzn Forsch* 1976 28, found vinpocetine helped inhibit platelet aggregation to blood vessels of the eye in a study of 100 patients.

Wollschlaegger, *J Am Nat Assoc* 2001 4:2 looked at 39 articles written on vinpocetine over the years. One of three met proper methodology, according to the author leaving a total of 327 patients with the drug or placebo in selected clinical trials. Statistically significant improvement in cognitive function and memory was noted.

Vinpocetine may be useful in the phase between mild cognitive impairment and the development of senile dementia or Alzheimer's disease; at least slowing the disease process and decreasing the incidence. Vinpocetine is, however, ineffective in improving cognitive function in those patients suffering the disease.

Studies have shown antioxidant activity equivalent to vitamin E.

Vinpocetine may be of help in protecting from the after effects of ischemic stroke, at least in one randomized clinical trial.

In a multi-centre, double-blind, placebo-controlled study of 203 patients suffering mild to moderate psycho-syndromes, including primary dementia, significant improvement was found after 16 weeks.

In Russia, vincamine is prepared with methanol to produce a drug called Metvin. This product possesses a ganglion-blocking action, accompanied by a dilatation of the blood vessels, and a fall in arterial pressure. It is recommended for medical practice in that country.

Vintoperol is another derivative of vincamine that enhances blood flow to the lower extremities, but has toxic side effects.

Vasicine possesses cerebral stimulating properties.

The leaves and stems of *V. minor* and *V. variegata* have been studied in Iran, for their inhibitory effect on *Leishmania major.*

Studies by Bojthe et al have shown plants fed tryptophan, tryptamine or lysine contain many more alkaloids (vincamin, vincin, vinaminin, vincinin), especially in young shoots.

Tryptophan and lysine together caused an unexpected drop in alkaloid content.

The LD 50 for vincamine in mice is 1000 mg/kg, about one-third the toxicity of caffeine.

The plant contains the indoles, resperine and reserpinine. The former is a monamine transporter, and vesicular monamine transporter to the brain and adrenals, with anti-hypertensive, anti-psychotic, tranquilizing, neuroleptic CNS anti-depressant activity.

Reserpinine is a VMT transporter as well. Both names are commonly associated with the medicinal herb *Rauwolfia serpentina,* or Indian Snakeroot, long prized for anti-depressant and hypotensive activity.

HOMEOPATHY

Vinca minor (Lesser Periwinkle) is considered a useful remedy for various skin conditions like eczema of the head and face.

There is a great sensitivity of the skin, with redness and soreness from slight rubbing (corrosive itching).

The scalp can have itching, or bald spots; with oozing moisture that mats the hair.

The individual may suffer whirling vertigo, and have a ringing or whistling in the ears.

The nose is red on tip, with sores and stoppage in one nostril. Seborrhea on the upper lip and base of nose is common. Weeping inflammations of the upper respiratory passages, as well as nasal polyps indicate this remedy.

Passive, uterine hemorrhage between periods, or continuous, heavy and excessive menstruation; and hemorrhage from fibroids are all symptoms of its use.

Symptoms are worse after swallowing.

Mentally, the patient is cross, with quick temper but repentant soon afterward.

They may dream of being threatened and cursed by a patient that has been treated unsuccessfully.

There may be the sensation of insects or spider webs on face.

DOSE- First to third potency. The mother tincture is made from the fresh plant, gathered when coming into flower.

The original proving was down by Rosenberg on five provers with mother tincture in 1838. In 1893 a proving was conducted by Schier, on two females and six males with tincture, 2x, 6c, and 10c potencies.

GEMMOTHERAPY

Vinca minor is hypotensive and helps thin blood. It is useful for increasing circulation to the brain and relieving migraines associated with spasmodic conditions.

DOSE- 10-30 drops three times daily of glycerine macerate.

HYDROSOL

Periwinkle herb is distilled in May and the water is used for women with a cold womb or stomach. **BRUNSCHWIG**

FLOWER ESSENCES

Periwinkle (*V. minor*) flower essence helps one integrate personal philosophy and ideals with higher spiritual concepts.

The conscious, subconscious, and super conscious minds are linked; and some subconscious impulses may conflict with ideals. The person may be restless with their current status and are looking for a deeper meaning to life. **PEGASUS**

Periwinkle flower essence aids in clearing past life experiences which block the flower of energy to a particular organ. **PETITE FLEUR**

Periwinkle essence has a calming and balancing effect. It promotes "nerves of steel". **KORTE**

At the physical level, Periwinkle affects hypertension, hemorrhaging and nervous disorders especially anxiety states. It calms the mind. It is also used for SAD which is a type of depression caused by insufficient sunlight to stimulate the production of a hormone called melatonin during the winter months.

Periwinkle lifts the dark cloud of depression regardless of what apparently caused it. It moves us to the place of inner knowing, our place of deepest wisdom, where we remember who we are. **PACIFIC**

Vinca minor flower essence helps create strong nerves and lets us keep track under chaos. **MIRIANA**

PERSONALITY TRAITS

Perry Winkle's Paint Brush

The first Spring descended upon the earth, and…the view from the hilltop across mile after mile of wildflowers with all different blossom and leaf shapes revealed one startling, glaringly obvious thing. Somehow, the finishing touch had been overlooked! All the flowers were one color-White!

The very last flower to have been created was the humble periwinkle. Thus, he was the one called upon to solve the problem of coloring all of the flowers.

"Goodness, gracious" said Perry in a small, blue voice. "I am depressed. There is just no way a little flower like me could color all the flowers in the world."

"Perry," a deep, soft voice resounded, "what you need is a little faith! In this world everyone has a job and is expected to work. The job for you and your family will be to paint all the flowers every color to be found on our earth and in our sky."

"But how can I do such a thing? There are not enough brushes or paint in the world to color the millions of flowers you have strewn on this planet." Perry said in a defeated tone.

"The rainbow will be your never-ending supply of colors. And listen closely: Slip your petals off, and you will see that I have given every periwinkle in my kingdom its very own paintbrush." **LOVEJOY**

RECIPES

TINCTURE- LEAF AND ROOT- six drops up to three times daily. One part plant to five parts 45% alcohol for dry plant; 1:2 of fresh herb at 60%.

INFUSION- One ounce dried herb to one pint of boiling water. Infuse 15 minutes. Drink one half cup as needed.

VINCAMINE- 10-20 mg 3 times daily. It takes 3-6 weeks before subjective and objective improvements are noted.

VINPOCETINE- 10 mg three times daily. Bioavailability is improved 60-100% when taken with food, mainly absorbed via the small intestine. Absorption is as low as 7% on empty stomach.

CAUTION- Periwinkle is contra-indicated in low blood pressure. In excess, it can produce granulocytopenia and bone marrow depression. Do not use with brain tumours or acute brain injury, and due to a reduction in ability to clot, should be avoided by hemophiliacs and those taking anti-coagulants. Do not use during pregnancy.

PROPAGATION- By root divisions in the spring or fall. Propagation from cuttings, using a rooting hormone, works very well.

Space plants 15-20 inches apart. Prefers partial shade, but will do well in full sun.

HARVESTING- Microwave technology appears to be quite useful in drying medicinal herbs, with the majority of cases showing no negative effect to the pharmacological compounds. However, in one study by Kartnig et al, *Pharmazie* 1996 51:12 vincamine was the only substance altered by microwave (300-1200 watts) energy. In many cases, the microwaved herbs contained higher concentrations of determined constituents than the air dried herbs.

BELTED CAP PANAEOLUS
DARK RIMMED MOTTLEGILL
(*Panaeolus subbalteatus*)
(*P. cinctulus* [Botton] Saccardo**)**
(*P. venenosus*)
BELL CAP PANAEOLUS
PINCHED PANAEOLUS
HOOPED PETTICOAT
PETTICOAT MOTTLEGILL
(*P. campanulatus* [Bull,:Fr] Quél**)**
(*P. papilionaceus* [Bull,:Fr] Quél**)**
(*P. sphinctrinus* [Fr.] Quél**)**
(*P. retirugis* [Fr.] Quél**)**
PARTS USED – dried fruiting bodies

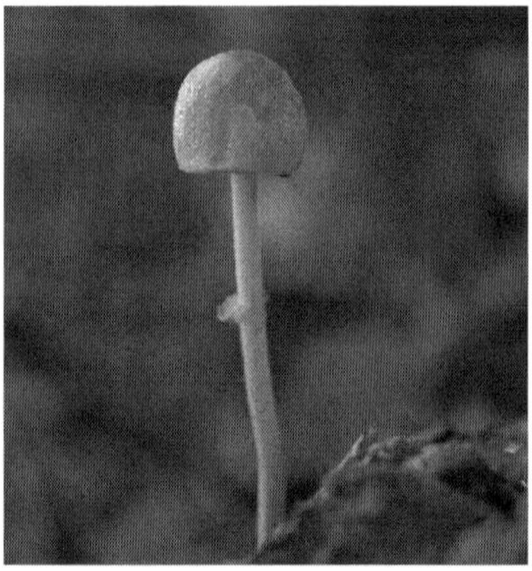

Panaeolus sphinctrinus

Panaeolus subbalteatus is the classic Druid mushroom.

DANIEL DELANEY

Horse Manure also has a chance in the time of giant mushrooms.

KOBAYASHI ISSA

Panaeolus is Greek meaning "all variegated or dazzling", while subbalteatus is Latin, meaning "darker border on cap". This is from the prefix sub meaning almost or somewhat, and balteatus, meaning belt-like, in reference to the darker color zonation that form along margins of the cap while drying.

Sphinctrinus is Greek meaning, "tied up or pulled in". Venenosus is based on a previous undeserved reputation of poisonous. Papilionaceus is from Papilo meaning a butterfly, as in the movie Papillon.

I have found Belted Cap Panaeolus growing on lawns in my home city of Edmonton. It is recognized by a dark, marginal band on the cap after which it is named. The spore print is black, the stem pinkish brown.

This common garden mushroom contains psilocybin (1.6-6.5 mg/gram dry wt), and baeocystin, but no psilocin (4-hydroxy-di-methyl-tryptamine).

Psilocybin, however, becomes psilocin in the body, after phosphorus is stripped away by enzymes. It contains large amounts of serotonin and 5 HTP (5-hydroxytryptophan).

Psilocin concentrates in higher amounts in the liver and adrenals, and in the brain of rats has been found to concentrate in the neocortex, hippocampus and thalamus.

This makes it a magic mushroom of the prairies with true psychotropic activity. One 34 year old Scot ingested over 20 fruit bodies, and experienced mild hallucinogenic reactions without nausea. Within one hour the sensations of detachment were experienced, followed by feelings of unmotivated hilarity.

It is considered more empathogenic and aphrodisiac than mushrooms that contain only psilocybin. Individual visions are observed for longer periods of time and contemplated at a leisurely pace, according to Christian Ratsch. As little as one and a half grams dry weight produce psychoactivity, while 2.7 grams are considered a visionary dose.

After a 40-year hiatus, psilocybin is again being researched for its benefit in addiction, schizophrenia, paranoia, and depression. Dr. Griffiths conducted a study of 36 adults and published results in July 2006 issue of the journal *Psychopharmacology*.

"It opens up the whole adventure in neuroscience to chart brain functions during mystical experiences", says the author.

Dr. David Nichols, at Purdue University, says that psilocybin and psilocin "are some of the most potent compounds we know of that can change consciousness. It's kind of peculiar they have just been kind of sitting on the shelf for 40 years. There is no other class of biologically active substances I am aware of that have been ignored like that".

The German name means Dark Banded Dung Mushroom, while the Japanese call it **MAGUSOTAKE**, or horse pasture mushroom. The mushroom does like horse ranches and similar environments.

Cochran and Lucas (1959) reported that *P. subbalteatus* provides significant protection from the polio virus in mice studies.

Psilocybin mushrooms might be of further use improving eyesight, hearing, circulation, and activating the self-healing processes within the human body.

Work by J. Gartz, in a publication of the *British Mycological Society*, suggests recent studies show psilocybin at low doses is effective against acute migraine and cluster headaches. It likely affects the serotonin receptor (5-HT) in a fashion analogous to Summertryptan, a drug used for this purpose. Some work in this area could yield a medicine that has low toxicity and few side effects for these debilitating conditions.

Spoerke and Rumack, in their excellent book, report that migraine headache patients were found to be more sensitive to the hallucinogenic effects of psilocybin in a placebo controlled study of 30 normal subjects and 36 migraine patients. After an oral dose of 20 mcg/kg, no reaction occurred in 86% of control compared to 41% of migraine patients. Hallucinations occurred in 18% of migraine patients and none in control.

Possible mechanisms for this increased sensitivity could be increased blood brain barrier permeability and/or CNS serotonin sensitivity.

Pinched Panaeolus, also common on prairies and the west coast has recently been reported to contain psilocybin, and serotonin, and is definitely a hallucinogen. It was used by the Mazatec and natives of Mexico, and known as She-to or To-shka.

She-to means “pasture mushroom”, and To-shka “intoxicating mushroom”. And while it is not as important as other species of the Psilocybe and Stropharia, various shamans have used it on occasion.

In China, the mushroom is known as **HSIAO CHUN**, or laughing mushroom.

A number of myths and works of art in ancient Greece depict Nessus, the Centaur, with a mushroom sprouting between his hooves. It may well been the fungal ambrosia associated with Eleusinian and Orphic mystery.

Jonathan Ott wrote than some individuals in Oregon take up to 250 specimens of this species in order to produce a strong hallucinogenic effect.

Pinched Panaeolus produces laccase isoenzymes and manganese peroxide with activity at high pH levels.

Bell Cap Panaeolus (*P. campanulatus*) contains psilocybin, but also ibotenic acid (like Amanita) that causes nausea. Not recommended. Work by Hervey in 1947 showed activity against *E. coli*.

The mushroom *P. papillonaceus* is part of the *P. campanulatus* complex. Work by Mukherjee and Sengupta, *Can J Microbiol* 1985 31:9 found this mushroom to be a high producer of inulinase and invertase at optimum pH of 6.5 at 60° C.

Mukherjee et al in India, *Current Microbiology* 27:1 has found this species resistant to nystatin and amphotercinin B.

The related, West Coast species, *P. retirugis,* contains the antibiotic diterpene, pleuromutilin in mycelical culture. Two new illudane sesquiterpenes, paneolic and paneolilludinic acid show activity against *Staphylococcus aureus*.

Paneolic acid exhibits cytotoxicity against HL60 cells with an IC50 of 18.9 mcg/ml. Ma et al, *J Antibiotics* (Tokyo) 2004 57:11.

HOMEOPATHY

P. campanulatus is related to memory loss and gain, reeling about, sudden dimness of vision, slow and feeble pulse, languor and weakness, giddiness, trembling and great drowsiness.

ALLEN'S ENCYCLOPEDIA - VERMEULEN

HAYMAKER'S MUSHROOM
BROWN HAY CAP
LAWN MOWER'S MUSHROOM

(*Panaeolina foenisecii*)
(*Panaeolus foenisecii*)
(*Psathyrella foenisecii*)

Panaeolina means small Panaeolus, and foenisecii literally dry hay, both from Latin. Psathyrella means fragile.

This small parasol mushroom is a common lawn mushroom. It has a dark purplish brown spore print, and fruits in summer on the western prairies.

Small amounts eaten raw are considered poisonous to young children, according to some authors.

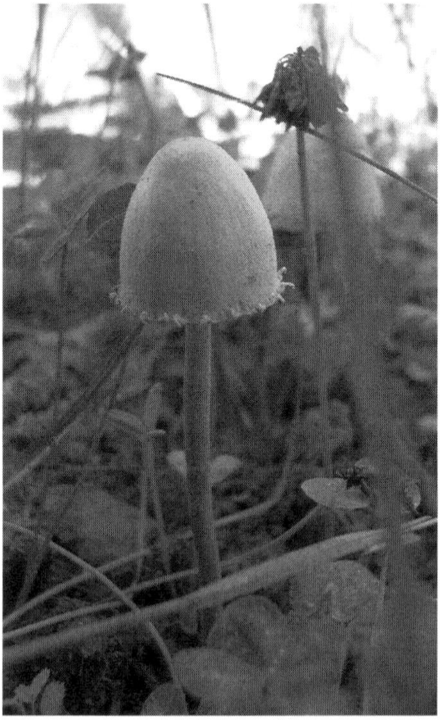

Bell Cap Panaeolus
(Courtesy of Paul Kroeger)

The mushroom contains psilocybin, according to some sources. Studies from Europe indicate no detectable psilocybin or its hallucinogenic derivatives, baeocystin and psilocin.

One study found 5-hydroxytryptamine (serotonin) and its precursor 5-hydroxytryptophan. In one test, forty grams of fresh mushroom failed to produce psychotropic effect.

Not all samples have been found to contain psilocybin.

Blue staining may or may not mean anything.

ROUND DUNG MUSHROOM
(*Psilocybe coprophila*)
(*Stropharia coprophila*)
(*Deconia coprophila* [Bull.] P Karst**)**
DUNG MUSHROOM
(*S. merdaria*)
(*P. merdaria* [Pers.:Fr] Kummer**)**
GARLAND STROPHARIA
(*P. coronilla* [Bull.:Fr] Noordel)
(*S. coronilla*)
HEMISPHERICAL STROPHARIA
ROUND DUNG HEAD
(*Protostrophia semiglobata* [Batsch] Redhead, Moncalvo & Vilgays**)**
(*S. semiglobata*)
(*S. semiglobata* var. *stercoraria*)
(*P. semilanceata* [Fr.] P. Kumm.**)**
LIBERTY CAP
PIXIE CAP
(*P. semilanceata*)
(*Panaeolus similanceata*)
BLUE GREEN STROPHARIA
VERDIGRIS TOADSTOOL
(*S. aeruginosa*)
(*P. aeruginosa* [Curtis:Fr.] Noor.**)**
(*Pratella aeruginosa*)

The little mushroom comes of itself, no one knows whence, like the wind that comes we know not whence nor why.**MAZATEC SAYING**

In my experience, psychedelic mushrooms, such as *Psilocybe semilanceata*…have the potential, if used carefully with knowledge and awareness, to be useful for developing sensitivity to the cycles of nature, to learn how we can be in harmony with its processes.
CHRISTOPHER HOBBS

Let us cheer for dung fungi!
Dung fungi —- unsung fungi!
Never-touch-the-tongue-fungi!
High-strung, ever-young fungi!
Freely flung across the dung
Freshly sprung with ho so gung!
Stench a song so plainly sung!

R. C. SUMMERBELL MYCELIUM April 1983

Psilocybe is from the Greek meaning bare head. Coprophila means dung loving. Merdaria is Latin, also pertaining to dung.

Stercoraria is derived from the minor Roman god Stercutus, the son of Faunus and the patron of manure. Liberty Cap is derived from the emblem worn by the figure of Liberté during and after the French Revolution. It is originally associated with the Phrygian bonnet.

The mushrooms are widespread and common, often found growing on manure.

Round Dung is one of the few Psilocybes on the Great Plains east of the Rockies. It contains low amounts of psilocybin, but no psilocin when fresh.

The mushroom shows activity against *Bacillus subtilis, S. aureus* and *E. coli.*

The body apparently hydrolyzes psilocybin, the indole alkaloids, into psilocin, the bioactive compound. The psychic activity is based on interference with the neurotransmitter, serotonin, which is structurally similar to psilocin. They are also closely related to DMT.

Psilocin binds to the serotonergic receptor, 5HT2a and acts as a partial agonist. That is, it stimulates some neurons and not others. The exact pathway to psychedelic experience is unknown, but one hypothesis is that an increased activity of the sensor motor gating system of the brain is involved. This system normally suppresses the majority of sensory stimuli from conscious awareness, so we can operate at a normal level.

The conscious mind is overwhelmed by sensory stimuli and cognitive processes normally hidden in the conscious part of the mind.

Liberty Cap is the most common West Coast "Magic Mushroom", and fruits during the rains of autumn. It has been found to inhibit *Staphylococcus aureus* bacteria.

In the early 1970s, I went with a friend and lined up all night for Rolling Stones tickets at the PNE in Vancouver. It was a great party, but alas no ticket in the morning as it was a sell-out. That evening we ventured down to Gastown and bought a large bag of fresh Liberty Caps.

We traveled up to Sechelt and made a mushroom omelet with our find. I remember the pleasant sensations of color and sound around me on the Pacific Ocean. I picked up a piece of driftwood and by late afternoon had carved a Polynesian style artwork, representing our male/female duality.

All species vary in their effects and due to variety of constituents may well react differently in individuals.

Paul Kroeger, one of British Columbia's finest mycologist, notes there are 10 Psilocybe species with hallucinogenic properties in that province.

Richard Haard, in Poisonous and Hallucinogenic Mushrooms, relates his experience with six different species of Psilocybe.

"*P. cyanescens* generally lets me look into the order which my inner mind forces on the rest of me; *P. semilanceata* is a model builder allowing me to look into the past, present and future of my life and activities, even into the very nature of life and eternity; *P. strictipes* and *P. baeocystis* both give a visual adventure, with baeocystis the most visual mushroom thus far."

P. cubensis is found around the Gulf of Mexico, and due to its size is often used for home and commercial growing.

There appears to great bias toward mushroom species containing psilocybin. It may surprise readers to find that research by Dr. Adrian North found 12.3% of opera music lovers have used magic mushrooms at one time or another. His research, published in the *Psychology of Music* 2007 35 journal involved 2500 people.

Charles Schuster, former director of the National Institute of Drug Abuse, notes a return to the study of certain hallucinatory compounds that showed potential into the nature of human consciousness and sensory perception.

"Human consciousness...is a function of the ebb and flow of neural impulses in various regions of the brain-the very substrate that drugs such as psilocybin act upon. Understanding what mediates these effects is clearly within the realm of neuroscience and deserves investigation."

A study conducted at Johns Hopkins found that 79% of subjects given psilocybin capsules under a controlled setting said the experience had changed them for the better.

Another study by Dr. Roland Griffiths is underway at the present time.

A news release from Reuters, dated July 3 2008, noted "the 'spiritual' effects of psilocybin from so-called sacred mushrooms last for more than a year. Griffiths et al, *J Psychopharm* 2008 22:6.

In 2006, Roland Griffiths and colleagues of John Hopkins University, gave synthetic psilocin to 36 volunteers and asked them how it felt. Most reported having a 'mystical' or 'spiritual' experience and rated it positively. "More than a year later, most still said the experience increased their sense of well-being or life satisfaction". Griffiths et al, *Psychopharm* (Berl) 2006 187:3.

In the same year, work by Sewell et al, *Neurology* 66 found the mushroom aborted cluster migraine headaches in 22 of 26 patients and 18 of 19 had extended remissions from the debilitating head pain.

Again in 2006, Moreno et al, *J Clin Psychol* 67 published a paper on the efficacy of psilocybe for OCD or obsessive-compulsive disorder, with positive results.

A study of psilocybin for treating schizophrenia was conducted by Vollenweider et al, *Neuropsychopharm* 2007 32:9.

Dr. Charles Grob of the Los Angeles Biomedical Research Institute is conducting a study to measure the effectiveness of psilocybin on the reduction of anxiety, depression and physical pain in stage IV cancer patients.

In 2009, Johns Hopkins began recruitment for a psilocybin study involving cancer patients.

A new study by British researchers has shown for the first time that psilocybin, which triggers feelings of oneness with the universe, works by reducing brain activity.

Under the influence of magic mushrooms, overall brain activity drops, particularly in parts associated with sensory areas. When functionally normally these connections appear to constrain the way we see, hear and experience the world, helping ground in "reality". These are the key nodes of brain linked to self-consciousness and depression. Psilocybin cuts activity to these nodes, severs connection to other brain area and allows the senses to run free.

Robin Carhart-Harris authored the study published in *Proceedings of the National Academy of Sciences* 2013. "The results seem to imply that a lot of brain activity is actually dedicated to keep the world very stable and ordinary and familiar and unsurprising.

Aldous Huxley, who explored entheogens in The Doors of Perception, predicted that many of the human brain's highest achievements involve preventing actions instead of initiating them, and sifting out useless information instead of collecting and presenting for conscious consideration. He coined the term psychedelic from the Greek psyche for mind, and delos for manifest.

The two areas of the brain showing greatest decline in activity were the medial prefrontal cortex and the posterior cingulate cortex.

The former, when dysfunctional is linked with rumination and obsessive thinking. In depression is it often overactive. The latter plays a key role in consciousness and self-identity, ego and personality. The dissolution of ego, reduction of selfishness and one with the universe helps bring profound peace.

They also found support for claims that sufferers of cluster headaches found reduced frequency of attacks. Over-activity in the hypothalamus is believed responsible, and psilocybin calmed this region of the brain.

A recent article in *Experimental Brain Research* 2013 228(4): 481-91 looked at effects of psilocybin on fear conditioning in mice. Authors suggest it should be further explored as a potential treatment of PTSD, or post-traumatic stress disorder. According to the PTSD Alliance, more than 13 million Americans suffer the condition at any given time.

Dung Mushroom is believed to contained small amounts of hallucinogenic compound by some authors. Paul Stamets suggests both are non-psilocybin species.

In Traditional Chinese Medicine, it is used to treat Kashin-Beck disease, and is one of the main components of Pine Mushroom Elixir. Kashin-Beck is a form of polyarthritis believed caused by eating grain contaminated with another fungus, *Fusarium sporotrichiella.*

Inhibition rate against sarcoma 180 is 80% and Erhlich carcinoma cancer cells 70%.

The tetraprenylphenol Suillin has been identified as the principle responsible for the mushrooms cytotoxic activity.

Round Dung Head grows on horse or cow dung in pastures and is identified by a bright yellow gel covering them when young. According to Arora, it is edible but slimy and mediocre.

In one experimenter, the mushroom caused dizziness, in-coordination, unprovoked hilarity, depression and space and time distortion. It does not stain blue.

Work by Alarcon et al, *Z Naturforsch* 2008 63 found this mushroom bio-transformed 5-hydroxytryptophan to 5-hydroxytryptamine.

Stropharia stercoraria is a variant of *S. semiglobata.* A small species, *P. angustispora*, grows on marmot and elk dung in the Cascade Mountains. It is psychoactive.

The related *S. coronilla* may contain psilocybin, but is of dubious edibility and may be considered poisonous. Two teenagers seeking a hallucinogenic experience, only received intense "bone pain" upon ingestion.

Some sources cite malaise, headache, ataxia, dizziness, vomiting, hallucinations and confusion.

Garland Stropharia is a litter decomposing basidiomycete that has been found capable of metabolizing and mineralizing benzopyrene. Manganese ions at 200 μM increased the effect by four and twelve times respectively. A study of 16 different polycyclic aromatic hydrocarbons found the higher molecular mass ones more easily converted. Steffen et al, *Appl Environ Microbiol* 2003 69:7.

Blue Green Stropharia or Psilocybin is common on the Pacific Northwest coast. It has a heavy layer of green slime that washes away to expose the ochre yellow cap. It has the distinct odor of fresh tomatoes, according to Helene Schalkwijk-Barendsen.

It has not caused any poisonings in North America, or at least none reported. I wouldn't bother.

It contains some interesting fats and lipids. Dembitsky et al, *Phytochem* 1992 31:3; 1993 34:4.

Early work suggests anti-tumor activity with inhibition of sarcoma 180 and Ehrlich carcinoma cells at 70% and 60% respectively.

Both water and ethanol extracts cause inhibition and excitation of impulse activity of neurons in the hippocampus stratum pyramidale region of the brain. Moldavan et al, *Ukray Botan Zhurnal* 2001 58:2.

The related *P. argentipes* has been studied and may have application for OCD, or obsessive-compulsive disorder. Matsushima et al, *Biosci Biotech Biochem* 2009 73:8.

The related *P. pelliculosa* and *P. stuntzii* are both weak to moderate psychoactive species common to the Pacific Northwest.

There are some 180 species of mushroom that contain psilocybin and/or psilocin, not all in the *Psilocybe* genus.

Greatest danger is mixing them up with other LBMs, or little brown mushrooms that are lookalike.

CAUTION- Do not combine with MAO inhibitors, or alcohol.

Recent work suggests that the content of psilocin can vary by up to 100 fold when grown in dark vs. light conditions. This is significant. Rafati et al, *Int J Med Mush* 2009 11:4.

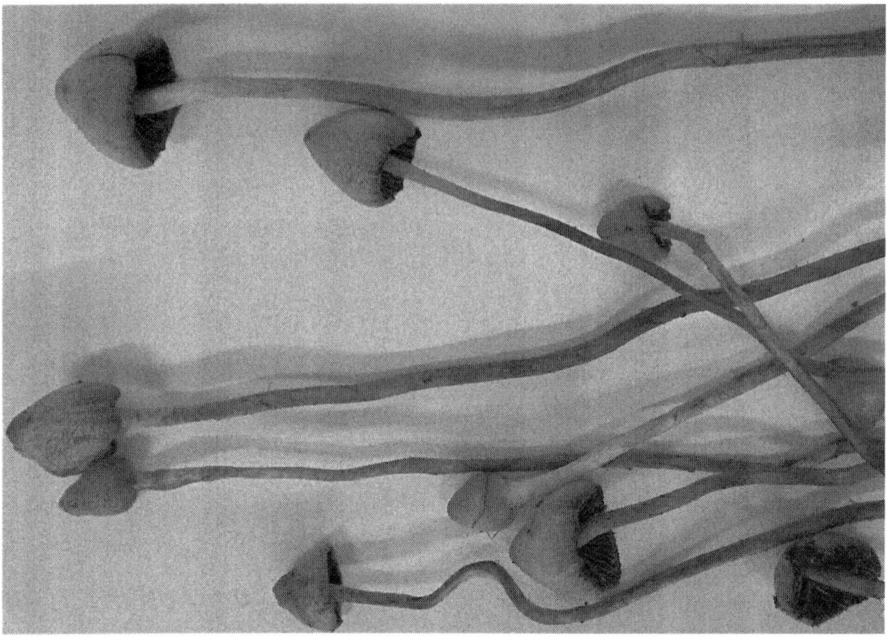

Panaeolus species

HOMEOPATHY

Absentminded when conversing, delusions of ants, changing suddenly, creative powers, alternately god and the devil, or in communication with God. Other delusions include possessing infinite knowledge, hearing beautiful music from primitive source, vertigo with blurred vision, head pain, drowsiness, metallic taste in mouth.

DOSE- A proving of *P. caerulescens* was carried out in 1968 by David Flores Toledo, using mother tincture, 5X, 6C, 12C, and 30C. A full record can be found in La Revue Belge d'homeopathie, 1984 36.

VERMEULEN

Psilocybe (*P. semilanceata*) is for symptoms of the mind including fear of death, euphoria, feelings of unreality, withdrawn and uncommunicative; obsessive compulsive behavior, distortion of time and space, numbness and tingling of limbs, dizziness, hyper-reflexia in deep tendon reflexes, dilated pupils, blurred vision, lively colors, increased auditory acuity, flushing of neck and face, yawning, incontinence, and temporary erythema-like chest eruptions.

DOSE- Low potency. This proving was by Bonnet et al, The toxicology of *P. semilanceata*, The Liberty Cap. *Homeopathic Links* 4/02. **VERMEULEN**

SPIRITUAL PROPERTIES

Henry Munn wrote a fascinating paper called The Mushrooms of Language. It may be found in Hallucinogens and Shamanism, Michael Harner Editor, Oxford University Press, 1973.

"Language is an ecstatic activity of signification. Intoxicated by the mushrooms, the fluency, the ease, the aptness of expression one becomes capable of are such that one is astounded by the words that issue forth from the contact of the intention of articulation with the matter of experience… The spontaneity the mushrooms liberate is not only perceptual, but linguistic, the spontaneity of speech, of fervent, lucid discourse, of the logos in activity. For the shaman, it is as if existence were uttering itself through him. **MUNN**

The principle gift of the psilocybin mushroom is that it allows one to commune directly with the vastly powerful intelligence that is located within all of Nature…With psilocybin-enhanced perception, I saw the trees without the usual mechanistic associations. They were no longer trees in the mundane sense, but something quite different. It was as if I were seeing for the very first time. And, once again, I was graced with the overall impression, the principal insight, that trees and plants are slowly moving organismic expressions of intelligence. Oaks manifest one kind of intelligence, pine trees another, but both are manifestations of natural intelligence….

I am convinced that the paradigm of natural intelligence, forged in me as a result of my numerous encounters with Nature's wilder side, could play a useful role in restoring our planet's health and healing our dysfunctional relationship with the rest of Nature…By encouraging extreme ecological sensitivity, psilocybin mushrooms may serve as a kind of medicinal antidote to the poisonous impact of rampant materialism.

At the least, the mushrooms can show us how we have severed ourselves from the natural system of intelligence that birthed us and that still sustains our existence. **SIMON G. POWELL**

Much to my surprise and occasional dismay, I was pulled into the heaviest psychic experience I have ever encountered. I was possessed by the mushroom spirit almost as if it sought to teach me a lesson. It now seems that I was drawn into a psychoanalysis, which allowed me to act out my personal conflicts by alternately becoming the conflicting selves and always observing myself at the same time.

Something had suddenly appeared out of the creative depths of my mind, something of which I was previously unaware. I underwent an awesome, fear-filled, but enlightening experience. Without respect you may be pulled into a vortex which you have no desire to enter. If you insist on stepping through the door of ecstasy, then prepare yourself with the writing of such people as John Lilly and Carlos Castaneda.

RICHARD HAARD

MYTHS AND LEGENDS

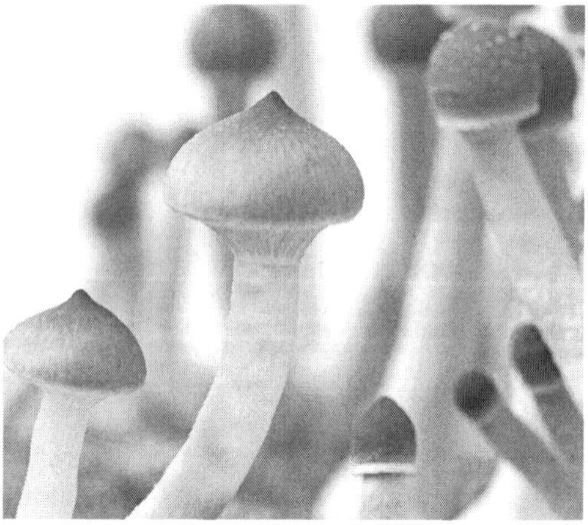

Magic mushroom

The fourth chapter of the Eiriks Saga Rautha gives a fairly detailed description of the woman named Lill-volvan, a "seeress" who travels from farm to farm predicting the future for the landowners. She was one of ten sisters who did this work. Unlike earlier Scandinavian shamanistic myths, this account is filled with intriguing mushroom motifs that are highly suggestive of Psilocybe mushroom metaphors.

The seeress is dressed in a very special way. She wears a blue cloak, jewels, and a headpiece of black lamb decorated with white cat skins, and she carries a staff. I would suggest not only that her outfit is clearly a shamanic ritual costume, but also that it serves as an entheogenic metaphor. To begin with, Lill-volvan wears a black and white fur cap. It may be merely coincidental, but the cap of … the most common and most potent of the Psilocybes found in Scandinavia- is frequently black and white, as well as furry looking.

The seeress also wears a blue mantle (or cloak), which immediately brings to mind the tendency of Psilocybe stems to turn blue when they are handled. Furthermore, she sits on a cushion of chicken feathers. When a mushroom is picked, one often sees white, downy material at its base, which is part of the mycelium…

It is stated that the seeress wears a belt with mushrooms hanging from it. Moreover, on her belt hangs a pouch in which she keeps a "magical substance" that she reportedly uses in order to go into trance. It is not difficult to imagine what this substance might be.

STEVEN LETO SHAMANS DRUM 2000 54

RECIPE- From 0.25 grams of dry mushrooms to 0.75 grams depending upon sensitivity of ingester. Up to 2 grams or more can be used by more experienced people.

Toxicity is very low. Therapeutic index is 641, compared to aspirin at 199 and nicotine at 21. This index is a ratio of the ED50, or effective dose in 50% of subjects vs. the LD50 that kills 50% of subjects.

NOTE: Psilocybin mushrooms have been declared illegal by a number of countries in the last while. These include Denmark in 2001, Japan in 2002, Britain in 2005, Ireland in 2006, and Holland in 2007. Another example of politics getting in the way of good science.

Some excellent work at Johns Hopkins may change all that very soon.

GARDEN SAGE
DALMATIAN SAGE
(*Salvia officinalis* L.)
BLUE SAGE
(*S. nemorosa* L.)
PARTS USED- leaf

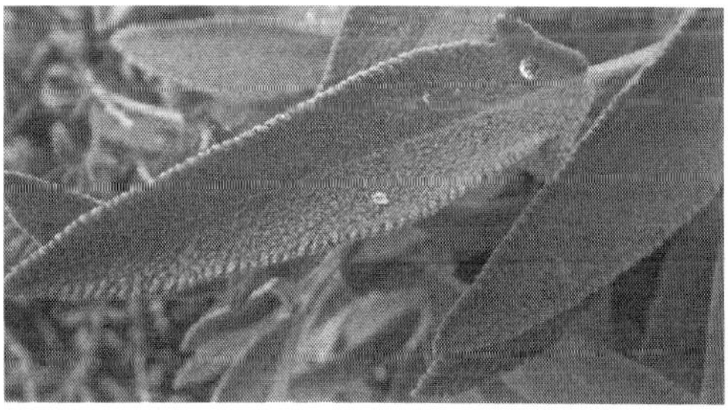

Common Sage

How can a man die who has sage in his garden?

ANCIENT PROVERB

He that would live for aye,
Must eat Sage in May.

ENGLISH PROVERB

Tis a plant endu'd with so many and wonderful properties, as that the assiduous use of it is said to render men Immortal. **JOHN EVELYN**

Salvia is from the Latin **SALVUS**, meaning to save, saviour or safe, and in turn from the Old Latin verb **SALVERE** meaning "to heal". It progressed to the Old French **SAUGE** and then to the English sage. Sage also relates to the word **SAPERE**, to taste, and of course, wisdom.

Officinalis refers to its official status as a medicine meaning "of the shop". Officina is a medieval word for shop or workshop, and source of the English office.

In Western Canada, common sage is an annual, often transplanted at 4-6 weeks from a greenhouse. It does occasionally survive a milder winter, but this event is rare. A pH soil from 6.2-6.4 is ideal. Work in Brooks, Alberta found that 80% of sage plants die without a protective winter mulch. Ouch!

Garden Sage is one of 900 species of Salvia wordwide, and yet is the one all others are measured against.

Parkinson, the famous English herbalist wrote in 1629: "Sage is much used of many in the month of May fasting, with butter and Parsley, and is held of most much to conduce to the health of mans body. It is also much used among other good herbes to be tunn'e up with ale, which thereupon is term'd Sage Ale, whereof many barrels full are made, and drunke in the said month chiefly for the purpose afore recited: and also for teeming women, to help them the better forward in the childebearing".

Sage ale was thought to be especially inebriating, according to Stephen Buhner. See recipe below.

In ancient Greece, returning soldiers were greeted, by their wives, with sage tea to stimulate fertility.

Gerard suggested that "sage is singularly good for the head and brain, it quickeneth the senses and memory, strengtheneth the sinews, restoreth health to those that have the palsy, and taketh away shakey trembling of the members".

Sage helps to flavour rich, fatty meat such as duck and goose, as well as pork.

Culpepper mentions the use of sage for treating hot flashes, a use still relevant today.

A 414 page book dedicated to sage was published in 1688 by the Danish doctor, Christian Paullini.

The Chinese, in past centuries, would trade black tea for sage, one pound of sage for three, with the Dutch.

In the Mediterranean, an insect bite from Cynips species induces a gall on the leaf much prized for eating. On the Greek Island of Zante, these galls are preserved in honey.

In Italy, sage is used to flavor veal, and browned butter for pasta dishes. Liver with sage is a popular dish in Venice, and used in pizza toppings. Germans and French chefs use the spice for cured meats, and the English made sage ale, and flavored cheese, mince pies and as an afternoon tea, long before the tradition of black tea.

Salvia officinalis was in the USP from 1842-1916 and in the *National Formulary* from 1936-1950. It is in the *British Herbal Pharmacopoeia* and *European Pharmacopoeia.*

Sage, thyme, peppermint and other herbs have been found a substitute for malachite green in preventing disease in aquaculture. *J Fish Aqua Sci* 2009 April 16.

Water extracts of sage show synergistic activity with various food grade preservatives such as sodium benzoate, potassium sorbate, and sodium nitrate. This suggests using less chemicals to accomplish preservation. Stanojevic et al, *Centr Eur J Biol* 5:4.

Blue or Wood Sage is a perennial herb introduced to the prairies, and found scattered along roadsides and waste grounds.

Blue Sage is related to the culinary cousin, with a similar fragrance to the leaves when crushed.

But it is hardier, and certainly a prettier plant with its beautiful, purple blooms that last all summer. It loves hot, dry and even alkaline soils, making it perfect for prairie conditions.

Recent perennial trials at the Calgary Zoo, found the plant had a 100% survival rate through several winters. Probably with mulch!

MEDICINAL

CONSTITUENTS- flavonoids, rosmarinic acid (3.5%), carnosol, carnosic acid (salvin), essential oils 1.5-2.5%, saponins, salvia tannin, caffeic acid trimers suh as melitric acid A, methyl melitrate A, sagecoumarin, salvianolic acid K, picrosalvin, salvin, labiatic and phenolic acids, ursolic acid, oleanolic acid, cis-p-coumaric acid, hydroxyluteolin, luteolin, vicenin-2, rosmanol, epirosmanol, guldosol, minerals, vit A and C.

Salvia tannins are not genuine tannins in the sense of condensed tannins or hydrolysable tannins. Carnosic acid readily oxidizes to carnosol and in turn produces genkwanin, hispidulin, cirsimaritin, and 5-methoxy-salvigenin.

S. nemorosa root- royleanones (diterpene phenanthrene- quinones)

aerial parts- 31 compounds including 41.6% beta caryophyllene, 21% germacrene B, 6.8% caryophyllene oxide, 6% cis-beta-farnesene, 5.6% germacrene D; nemorosin (deterpenoid) and salvinemorol (triterpenoid); salvionosides A, B, and C (megastigmane glycosides; (6S,9R)-and (6S,9R)-roseosides, (6R,9R)-and (6R,9S)-oxo-alpha-ionol glucosides, and blumeol C glycoside.

Sage is a stimulant, dry, warm astringent, tonic and carminative herb. It is very useful for stomach problems associated with weak digestion, and taken in the form of a warm, not hot, tea.

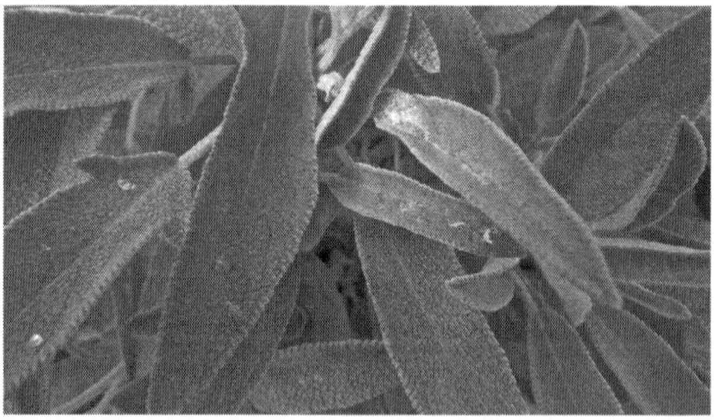

Garden Sage

Ethanol/water extracts of the herb show gastric protective activity, probably due in part to carnosol. Mayer et al, *Fitoterapia* 2009 80:7.

Hot sage tea helps at the onset of flu and colds, including fever, but the cold tea will decrease sweating, and mucus production of the nose, throat and lungs.

Sage is a very versatile herb. For insect bites, take a fresh leaf and crush or chew it, and apply it to the affected area. It will give quick benefit, but not as lasting as plantain.

A hot infusion with a little honey does wonders for a sore throat, loss of voice and tonsillitis in the form of a gargle.

A randomized, double-bind parallel studies of 286 patients with acute viral pharyngitis found a 15% sage extract spray was significantly better than placebo. Hubbert et al, *Eur J Med Res* 2006 11:1.

A sage/echinacea throat spray was compared to chlorhexidine/ lidocaine for treatment of acute sore throat. The herbal treatment was a little better during the first three days with both well tolerated. Schapowal et al, *Eur J Med Res* 2009 14:9.

It shows activity against vesicular stomatitis virus in work by Tada et al, Phytochem 1997 45; and inhibition of virus infective cycle. Smidling et al, *Arch Biol Sci* (Belgrade) 2008 60:3.

Relief from labial herpes was noted from an ointment containing sage and rhubarb. Saller et al, *Forsch Kompl Med Klass Naturheil* 2001 8.

Sage tea, taken warm, will help dry up a mother's milk supply, and help with the weaning process. It also dries up excessive salivation, and should be used with care in dry mouth conditions. Again, pay attention to the temperature it is used at.

In a number of open studies, sage has been found to reduce hyperhydrosis, a condition of excessive sweating. A 1980 unpublished study of 80 patients with idiopathic hyperhydrosis found excellent results.

Grieve mentioned the used of alfalfa and sage tea for menopausal hot flashes and night sweats. A study by De Leo V et al, *Minerva Ginecol* 1998 50:5 found a product of the two herbs improved hot flashes and night sweating in a three month open trial. It appears that the two herbs produce a slight anti-dopaminergic activity.

It will increase perspiration in those who do not sweat and dry up secretion in those who sweat a great deal; an amphoteric diaphoretic if you will.

A recent study of sixty-nine women average age of 56, menopausal for a year and at least five flushes daily found a single tablet of fresh sage significantly decreased episodes. After four weeks, half noted improvement and after 8 weeks 64% found reduction in numbers and severity of flushes. Bomner S et al, *Adv Ther* 2011 28:6.

A strong infusion will often relieve or clear nervous headaches.

A remedy for skin itching from the Bahamas involves decocting fresh leaves for about an hour and then bathing the afflicted area. A sprinkle of whole-wheat flour is applied and left to dry. A double blind randomized, placebo controlled study compared sage extract (2%) with 1% hydrocortisone, 0.1% betamethasone control, placebo or no treatment on erythema on backs of 40 human volunteers. The sage extract significantly reduces erythema compared to placebo and to similar extent as hydrocortisone. Reuter J et al, *Planta Med* 2007 73:11.

Sage tea is used as a hair rinse, both to darken and to improve both texture and tone of the hair.

Sage leaf can be smoked for asthma, as well as acute and chronic bronchitis.

Sage is much prized for its ability to relieve hot flashes associated with peri- and menopausal stages of life. Night sweats are particularly relieved, not only in the crone, but also in tubercular patients.

There is a drying of the skin and tendons associated with menopause or andropause.

Phyllis Light says it is a specific for the transition from fertility levels of estrogen to post-menopausal levels.

Sage also addresses infertility, and amenorrhea or scanty periods associated with uterine blood deficiency. It helps promote a difficult or slow to progress labour.

The herb's essential oils affect the pituitary, adrenals and gonads, as well as enhance non-specific immune function.

Research suggests its use in helping to lower blood sugar levels. This makes sense, as the adrenals take over the role of manufacturing small amounts of hormones after the gonads atrophy.

Work by Eldi et al, *J Ethnopharm* 2005 100:3 found the plant extract significantly lowered serum glucose in mild diabetic model. Lima et al, *Br J Nutr* 2000 96:2 found both the tea and essential oil resemble metformin in work on rat hepatocytes.

Peter Holmes compares it to schisandra berry as it "addresses chronic immune deficiency with recurring or chronic infections, and cerebral/systemic nervous deficiency with signs of mental deterioration, chronic fatigue, insomnia, etc."

It was used traditionally for fevers with lethargy and delirium, as well as restlessness and muscle spasms associated with low, prostrating fevers.

Note that the cold tea reduces sweating and the hot tea is a strong diaphoretic. Dr. Anthony Godfrey, a well-known naturopath in Toronto, says that sage "regulates virtually all fluids—blood, lymph, milk, sweat, urine—to maintain a healthy balance."

Do not use when night sweats are created by hectic fever and dry, harsh skin. Instead, think of excessive sweating associated with soft relaxed skin, cold hands and feet which sweat.

Sweating due to damp heat, night sweats and spontaneous sweating all call for cool tea. For genital itching, flatulence and other lower burner conditions, it helps dry dampness and cool heat. It combines well with Oregon grape root for these purposes.

Sage helps resolve chronic mucus conditions of the nose, including rhinitis, sinusitis, postnasal drip, and congestion due to its bitter and acrid nature.

Chronic, spasmodic asthma, associated with thick phlegm and wheezing, benefit from sage.

The sweet, aromatic and slightly bitter tea is useful for gastritis, colic, chronic diarrhea, mucous colitis and the like.

Sage tincture is gastro-protective, and helps reduce gastric secretions, possibly due to carnasol content. Mayer et al, *Fitoterapia* 2009 May 28.

The herb shows activity against both *Helicobacter pylori* and *Campylobacter* organisms. Cwikla et al, *Phytother Res* 2009 2003. Other herbs with activity against the former were agrimony and meadowsweet, and against the latter calendula, chamomile, fennel and milk thistle.

A combination of sage ethyl acetate or acetone extract and amoxicillin showed potent synergy against various antibiotic resistant bacteria from two to ten fold. Ethyl acetate extract showed synergy with chloramphenicol. Stefanovic et al, *Acta Pol Pharm* 2012 69:3 457-63.

Work by Lima et al, *Chem Biol Interact* 2007 167:2 found both water and methanol extract protect HepG2 cell lines.

It is a significant inhibitor of SW480 colon cancer cell growth. Yi et al, *J Sc Food Agric* 2011 91:10 1849-54.

It relieves urethritis, cystitis and clear vaginal discharges associated with damp, cold conditions.

A tincture of sage has been found to exhibit anti-inflammatory activity by reduction of marrow acute phase response and NO synthesis. Oniga et al, *Rev Med Chir Soc Med Nat Iasi* 2007 111:1.

Carnosic acid and carnosol are highly anti-inflammatory, and activate peroxisome proliferator-activated receptor gamma.

Sage relieves pain and is anti-inflammatory, possibly by modulating TRPA-1 receptors. Melissa Rodrigues et al, *J Ethnopharm* 2012 139:2 519-26.

Sage is phyto-estrogenic in nature, with anti-gonadotrophic activity, but with nervous system and adrenal cortex stimulating effect.

A recent double blind study found 150 mg capsules of sage taken three times daily decreased hot flashes in menopausal women. *Phytotherapy* 2012 26:2 208-13.

Chris Hedley suggests that sage taken internally and as a compress will soothe painful, lumpy breasts.

It helps promote clear thinking, absent-mindedness and depression associated with long- term fatigue.

This makes it useful in impotence and frigidity, as well as intermittent fevers, and autoimmune conditions due to its balancing effect of the five organ systems.

It is anti-spasmodic in action, as well as a vascular analeptic and gram-positive anti-bacterial. Brantner and Grein, *J Ethnopharm* 1994 44:1.

Sage extracts inhibit lipid peroxidation, due to the content of carnosol, rosmanol and carnosic acid. Hohman et al, *Planta Med* 1999 65:6; Wang et al, *J Nat Prod* 1999 62:3.

Celik et al, *Nat Prod Res* 2008 22:1, found sage water infusions a powerful anti-oxidant against trichloracetic acid, showing increased catalase and SOD in brain, liver and kidney after 50 days.

This anti-oxidant property lends itself to food preservation, suppression of fish odors, etc.

Hypotensive and spasmolytic activity have been confirmed in animal studies by Todorov et al, *Acta Physiol Pharm Bulg* 1984 10:2.

Sage contains, according to James Duke, six anti-inflammatory compounds, and may be useful in conditions such as carpal tunnel syndrome.

He suggests its use internally and as a douche for *Candida albicans*.

Ursolic acid was found to compose 50% of a chloroform extract and possess anti-inflammatory activity twice as potent as indomethacin. Baricevic et al, *J Ethnopharm* 2001 75.

Sage herb and essential oil inhibit acetylcholinesterase *in vitro*. Perry et al, *Int J Geriatr Psych* 1996 11:12. This suggests a use in prevention or treatment of Alzheimer's disease.

A study by Alchondzadeh et al, *J Clin Pharm & Ther* 2003 28:1 in a double-blind, randomized, placebo-controlled trial over four months found that sage significantly reduced agitation in patients with mild to moderate Alzheimer's disease. Improved scores on the Clinical Dementia Rating and the Alzheimer's disease Assessment Scale were noted.

Work by Kennedy et al, *Neuropsychopharmacology* 2006 31 identified cholinesterase inhibition in a trial of 30 patients in a double-blind, placebo controlled cross-over study. Mood and cognitive performance were improved with lower doses reducing anxiety and higher doses increasing alertness, calmness and contentedness on the Bond-Lader scales.

A recent study of twenty seniors over 65 years of age, found that a daily dose of 333 mg of sage was associated with significant enhancement of memory and improvement in accuracy testing. Scholey et al, *Psychopharm* 2008 198:127-39.

Work by Rutherford et al, *Neurosci Lett* 1992 35:2 identified diterpenes in sage that interact with the GABA-benzodiazepine receptors.

Several studies have noted improvement in memory, but also mood. Calm, and more alert for up to six hours after taking sage, may be related not just to blockage of cholinesterase but activity on cholinergic receptors and damping down brain inflammation.

Sage's dry and astringent properties are increased with longer infusion or decoction times. The trade off is reduced essential oil content.

Sage possesses anti-viral activity against both herpes simplex 1 and 2 from a 20% ethanol extract. Schnitzier et al, *Phytomed* 2008 15:1-2.

The herb as well as the isolated compounds oleanolic and ursolic acid, have been found active against vancomycin resistant *Enterococci bacterium* and *Streptococcus pneumoniae.* Carnosol and carnosic acid have been found synergistic with gentamycin against methicillin resistant *Staphylococcus aureus*. Horiuchi et al, *Biol Pharm Bull* 2007 30:6.

Carnosic acid, also found in Rosemary, increases glutathione levels *in vivo*, and protects against ischemial middle cerebral artery and reperfusion brain damage. Satoh et al, *J Neurochem* 2008 104:4. Work by Snowden R et al, *J Altern Complement Med* 2014 Mar 17 found sage highly effective against staph cultures.

Carnosic acid may be of benefit in oral cancers due to anti-lipid peroxidation and moderate carcinogenic detoxifying enzymes.

Carnosic acid may be a useful adjunct with arsenic trioxide for HL-60 human myeloid leukemia. It works via modulation of the PTEN/Akt signaling pathway inducing apoptosis with G1 arrest. Wang et al, *Chin J Integr Med* 2012 18:12 934-41.

Matthew Wood has noted its use to remove coagulated blood. He gives an example of a woman with hemangioma with dark, prominent unsightly veins that were greatly reduced with external use of sage.

The Nippon Roche Research Center in Kamakura, Japan has found that sage tea helps prevent blood clots from forming.

Sage also lowered total cholesterol, triglycerides, LDL and VLDL in a DB PC trial of 57 hyper-lipidemic patients taking 500 mg capsules three times daily versus placebo. Kimbakht et al, *Phytother Res* 2011 25:12.

Sage may have some benefit in preventing cancer formation. Jedinak et al, *Z Naturforsch* 2006 61:1-2 found beta ursolic acid inhibits urokinase and cathespin B protease. This results in an anti-metastatic activity against beta 16 melanoma cell lines.

Sage extracts induce apoptosis in two human colon cancer cell lines through inhibition of MAPK/ERK pathways. Xavier et al, *Nutr Cancer* 2009 61:4.

Earlier work by Radtke et al in same journal 58 found sage phenolics immune modulating with TNF, interleukin 6 and interferon like activity.

Yi et al, *J Sci Food Agri* 2011 March 30 found inhibition of human colon cancer cell lines at low doses.

Ethanol extracts show therapeutic or preventative action on angiogenesis in both *in vitro* and *in vivo* studies by Keshavarz et al, *Phytother Res* 2010 24:10.

The essential oil contains thujone, and combined with its uterine stimulating properties, makes sage contraindicated during pregnancy.

Sage may interact with certain drugs, due to phase 1 enzyme interactions. Lima et al, *Food Chem Tox* 2007 45:3.

Studies by Zupko et al, *Planta Medica* 2001 67:4 found 50% methanol extracts of Blue Sage as effective an antioxidant as Garden Sage (*S. officinalis*).

HOMEOPATHY

Sage controls excessive sweating when circulation is enfeebled. It also works with night sweats and with tickling coughs. It exerts a tonic influence on the skin.

DOSE- Tincture in 20 drop doses in water.

ESSENTIAL OIL

CONSTITUENTS- linalyl acetate, geranyl acetate, oxides, alpha thujone (12-35%) and beta thujone (2-33%), camphor (5-20%), borneol 8%, linalool, geraniol, alpha bisabol, germacrene D, limonene, alpha and beta pinene, mycrene, beta caryophyllene, alpha terpineol, junerol, alpha humulene, salvene, p-cymene, 1,8-cineole (2-15%).

Sage oil possesses analgesic, anti-fungal, anti-spasmodic, anti-viral, and mucolytic properties.

It has a wide range of uses including cellulite, due to its ability to dissolve lipids.

It may be taken in small doses internally for disinfecting the intestinal tract and helping restore normal bowel flora.

Like the herb, sage oil promotes hormonal production of adrenaline and noradrenalin from the medulla of the adrenal gland. It also has a positive benefit on the corium layer of the skin, helping influence estrogenic and water retaining properties via the stimulating effect on the adrenal cortex. It helps improve the health of the skin during and after menopause. Work by Dr. Gumbel explains it well in greater detail.

Its activity is probably higher up, in the hypothalamus or pituitary. It reduces appetite, sexual desire and lactation all controlled by the master gland.

Work by Dorman and Deans, *J App Microbio* 2000 88:2 found the essential oil effective against *Staphylococcus aureus, E. coli* and *S. epidermidis.*

It is also anti-microbial against various *Salmonella species, Shigella sonnei, Klebsiella ozanae, Bacillus subtilis, Candida albicans* and *Cryptococcus neoformans.* Recio et al, Phytother Res 1989 3:77.

Work by Abravesh et al, *Iran J Med Arom Plants Res* 2005 20:4 add *Bacillus anthracis* and *B. cereus* to this list.

A study by Pereira et al, Rev Saude Publica 2004 38 showed 100% inhibition of *Klebsiella* and *Enterobacter* species, 96% inhibition of *E. coli,* 83% of *Proteus mirabilis*, and 75% inhibition of *Morganella morganii.*

Recent work found sage oil destroyed 72% of microbes within first hour and 70% reduction after 24 hours. Bonaziz et al, *Food Chem Tox* 2009 August 12.

Sage oil showed activity against species of *Klebsiella, Proteus, Escherichia, Staphylococcus, Streptococcus, Enterococcus, Enterobacter, Citrobacter* and *Acinetobacter* species in range of 0.78-25 ul/ml. Mihajilov-Krstev et al, *Centr Eur J Bio* 4:3.

Sage oil may be useful as a neurotonic in cases of alopecia, vertigo and general debility.

The essential oil was superior to control in a human trial of inhalation related to memory retention. Moss et al, *Human Psychopharm Clin &* Exp 25:5.

The undiluted oil on skin tests shows no irritation or allergic sensitization. Opdyke et al, *Food & Cosmetics Toxicology* 1976 14 supp.

CAUTION is advised for epileptics.

The oil is used in mouthwash, toothpaste, soaps, shampoo, detergents, anti-perspiration products, perfumes, soft drinks, and alcoholic beverages such as vermouth.

Sage oil shows activity against squamous carcinoma cells in oral cavity, suggesting a treatment for early stage mouth cancers. Sertel et al, *HNO* 2011 59:12 1203-8. Hydrosols may be good preventative gargle.

Blue sage is not presently grown on the prairies for its essential oil content. It does, however, have some potential, due to its hardy nature, and that its ketone content is less than *S. officinalis,* and its alcohol content, particularly borneol, much greater.

HYDROSOLS

Sage hydrosol contains 50-55% eucalyptol, 37-50% ketones, and 5-6% alcohols.

Viaud regards the hydrolat as an emmenagogue and relieves pelvic congestion.

Suzanne Catty considers the hydrosol to be one of the best lymphatic stimulants and cleanser.

She finds it a good hormonal balancer that helps regulate the menstrual cycle and relieve PMS and menopausal symptoms.

It also is excellent anti-wrinkle and anti-aging skin conditioner.

Sage hydrosol will raise blood pressure significantly more than essential oil. Caution is advised, according to Catty. Avoid during pregnancy.

Distil Sage whilst the flower be on it, the water strengthens the brain, provokes the menses, helps nature much in all its actions.

CULPEPPER

FLOWER ESSENCE

Sage flower essence is about drawing wisdom from life experience; reviewing and surveying one's life process from a higher perspective. Through Sage, the soul comes more in touch with its own spiritual meaning and purpose, and thus acquires profound wisdom to heal and counsel others. **FLOWER ESSENCE SOCIETY**

PERSONALITY TRAITS

Mature in age, which does not necessarily signified advanced in years, prompted by a certain wisdom and authority, she (Sage) addresses women, appealing more to their intelligence than their hearts. *Salvia officinalis* exerts her rigour against the tide in these times of emotional crisis where sexuality triumphs over conscience and love; she herself was earlier able to go beyond her troubles and sufferings, her crises and emotional illusions, which she skillfully turned to account to build up her exceptional character.

Associated more with inner than outer beauty, she affords women balance in their sex life by leading them towards a better understanding of their gynecological functions and what the feminine nature implies from the physical, as well as the psychic, point of view.

Tenacious, persistent, concise and efficient, she is socially a capable woman who is not afraid to impose her authority and strictness.

MAILHEBIAU

I've always felt rather sorry for garden sage. When the other plants are at their height of bloom and color, there sage sits, looking rather dowdy and plain, with its "army green" leaves…I think sage has come to terms with the fact that it's never going to be the bell of the ball. It faithfully returns year after year, happy to lend medicinal hand or content to simply stand in your garden and take a backseat to other more attractive herbs. Because of this, whenever I see garden sage, I always go over and say "hello". Funny thing is, it always thinks I'm talking to the plant behind it. **DEWEY**

For magical purposes the leaves are best harvested before the flowers appear. It's believed that if you can eat Sage in May, you will live a long life.

Carrying Sage on your person will encourage wisdom and help you connect with your intuition. **TRADITIONAL**

There is the very front glows sage, sweetly scented. It deserves to grow green forever, enjoying perpetual youth, for it is rich in virtue and good to mix in a potion of proven use for many a human ailment. But within itself is the germ of civil war, for unless the new growth is cut away, it turns savagely on its parent and chokes to death the older stem in bitter jealousy.

WALAHFRID STRABO
9TH CENTURY GERMAN MONK & HERBALIST

DOCTRINE OF SIGNATURES

The network of intricate, pebbly veins on the leaves resemble the small bumps on the tongue. The soft, velvety, hairy leaves, small than but similar to mullein leaves, call to mind the soft hairs lining the mucous membranes. The deep throated two-lipped flowers look like an open mouth with lips and tongue. These signatures significantly relate to the mouth and throat. If you put a leaf in your mouth and breathe in, you will feel a cooling sensation in your throat and then a warming feeling. It also has a drying effect.

These signatures, as well as the hint of bluish color in the flowers, also relate to the throat chakra and the mode of expression through communication of voice and sound.

The violet-purplish color of the flower corresponds to the brow chakra, which is linked to the pituitary gland, the endocrine system, and the corpus callosum that unites and balances the two hemispheres of the brain. The male and female symbolism of the flower also suggests balance.

The pungent, bitter taste of the plant is a signature of how deeply affected we can be by our own bitterness, which causes personal setbacks, lack of direction, the inability to manifest, and, most importantly, a lack of spiritual guidance and spiritual inspiration.

The white streaks in the flower are associated with the seventh chakra and imply purification, stabilization, and cleansing of the entire energy system. **PALLASDOWNEY**

ASTROLOGY

Sage is a remedy of the fifth chakra—the throat chakra. The throat and respiratory organs come under the dominion of Mercury, and the moon governs the brain and memory.

In addition to healing the lungs and throat, Mercury also governs active intelligence, analytical intellect, and reasoning powers. The moon represents awareness, sensitivity, receptivity, memory and imagination. Speech, writing, and communication are Hermetic gifts found in teachers, speakers, actors and singers—all of whom suffer one time or another from throat problems due to inhibition of the fifth chakra, or they suffer simply from overuse of the voice. In individuals, the influence of Mercury helps to bring a sense of rational balance to the moon propensity for suspicious, instinctive, confused behavior. With the positive gifts of imagination, memory and sympathy, the moon balances Mercury's tendency towards impatience, criticism and over-rationality. **GOODRICK-CLARKE**

RECIPES

TINCTURE- Fresh plant tincture prepared at 1:2 and 60% alcohol. 1-3 ml as needed. Do not use for long periods of time or during lactation unless there is a desire to wean.

ALE- Bring 4 gallons of water to boil, and add two ounces of fresh sage and two ounces of licorice root, simmer one hour. Cool to 160° F, strain over four pounds of malt extract and two pounds of brown sugar in fermenting vessel, stirring well.

Cool to 70° F and add yeast and two more ounces of fresh sage. Ferment for about a week. Bottle with one half teaspoon of sugar to each bottle and cap. Ready in 10-14 days. **STEPHEN BUHNER**

SALAD BURNET
GARDEN BURNET
(*Sanguisorba minor* Scop.)
(*S. minor subsp. minor*)
(*S. dictyocarpa*)
(*Poterium sanquisorba*)
COMMON BURNET
GREATER BURNET
ITALIAN PIMPERNEL
(*S. officinalis* L.)
(*S. polygama*)
(*P. officinale*)
SITKA BURNET
(*S. sitchensis* C. A. Mey)
(*S. stipulata*)
CANADA BURNET
(*S. canadensis* L.)
PARTS USED- leaves, root, flowers

It has two little leaves like unto the wings of birdes, standing out as the bird setteth her wings when she intendeth to flye. Ye Dutchmen calle it Hergottes Berdlen, that is "God's little birds", because of the colour that it hath in the topp. **WM TURNER 1551**

Salad is neither good nor beautiful
Where there is no pimpernella. **OLD PROVERB**

A salad without pimpernella is like love without a girl.
ITALIAN SAYING

Sanguisorba is from the Latin **SANGUIS**, meaning blood, and **SORBEO**, to absorb or **SORBERE**, to soak up, in reference to the hemostatic properties of the plant. Poterium is from the Greek **POTERION**, a drinking cup.

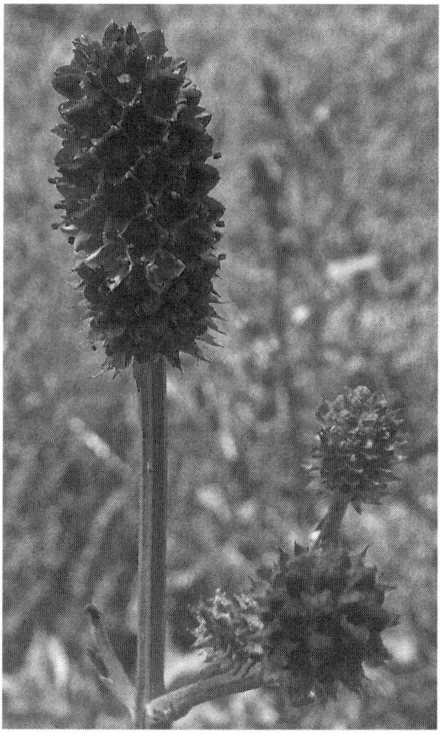
Common Burnet

Burnet is from the Old French, **BURNETTE**, or **BRUNETE** meaning dark brown, like the hair colour. Pimpernel is from the Old French **PIMPERNELLE**, descended from the Latin **PIPERINUS**, pepper-like. This alluded to Burnet's fruit, which was the old English name of Burnet. For some reason this was applied to Scarlet Pimpernel (*Anagallis arvensis*).

Common Burnet is a circumpolar plant found throughout the north from Alaska, and the Yukon, down into British Columbia and the northern prairies.

Salad, or Garden Burnet is naturalized from Eurasia, and both plants have been cultivated in gardens since the 1500s. Both are hardy to zone 3, at least.

In fact, I found Salad Burnet fresh herb at a market in northern Peru. It was sold for a salad or made into a tea for menstrual regulation.

They should not be confused with Burnet Saxifrage (*Pimpinella saxifraga*), a cultivated herb related to Anise. These are members of the rose family, revealed by the tiny compact five petal pink-green flowers.

The leaves have a fresh astringent bite, with a flavour like green walnut or cucumber, or both together. Older leaves are bitter and unpleasant.

Add to salads, ice drinks, vinegar, butter and cream cheese.

In parts of Japan and China, the leaves are preserved in salt as a type of pickle, or steamed when fresh.

In medieval times, the leaves were used to stop the flow of blood from wounds, and applied to sores, burns and cankers.

It was often combined with other herbs to treat diarrhea, dysentery, and other bowel disorders including ulcerative colitis. Excessive or abnormal menstrual bleeding also is relieved.

The 16th century herbalist, Turner suggested in one text that the leaves reminded him of a bird's wings in flight.

Pechy, in 18th century, felt Burnet was useful as one of 21 herbs in his anti-plague white wine mixture.

Culpepper wrote of Greater Burnet.

"This is an herb the Sun challenges dominion over and is a most precious herb, little inferior to Betony; the continual use of it preserves the body in health and the spirits in vigour; for if the Sun be the preserver of life under God, his herbs are the best in the world to do it by."

The English herbalist, Parkinson, wrote, "the greatest use that Burnet is commonly put unto, is to put a few leaves into a cup with Claret wine, which is presently to be drunke, and giveth a pleasant taste there unto, very delightful to the palate, and is accounted a help to make the heart merrie."

Greater Burnet has been used in traditional medicine for various internal bleeding conditions. Other uses include headaches, night blindness, hypertension and angina pectoris.

Salad Burnet-flavored wine has been used to treat gout and rheumatism.

John Evelyn wrote the "pimpernel eaten by the French and Italians, is our common Burnet; of so chearing and exhilerating a quality, and so generally commended."

Iroe Grego, in his unusual book, advised that the sword of a magician be bathed in the blood of a mole and the juice of Pimpinella.

Even Francis Bacon enjoyed the scent, and encouraged gardeners to cultivate it, "to perfume the air most delightfully, being trodden on and crushed."

Salad Burnet is the more familiar potherb used to flavour soups, cheese and salads. It has a cucumber-like taste, and is best used fresh in food.

The name suggests use in salads, but due to the tough nature of the leaves, it is best chopped fine in coleslaw, as a garnish, or integrated into a dressing.

One recipe that sounds tasty is to stuff a Cornish hen with burnet and lemons before roasting.

Root decoctions were traditionally used for skin burns. At one time, due to the tannins and astringency of the roots, it was used to tan leather a deep black.

Common Burnet is widespread throughout the Ural Mountains of Russia. The content of tanning substances was found highest in roots growing in grey wooded soils, and higher yet in forests.

An oil extracted from roots is used for burns, as well as pruritis, eczema and insect bites. The plant exhibits anti-tyrosinase and UV absorption activity, suggesting a use in reducing melanin pigmentation.

The leaves repel water, and when submerged in water, tiny air bubbles adhere to the surface, looking quite metallic and magical.

Work by Ushiki et al, *Soil Science and Plant Nutrition* 1996 42:2 found root extracts from Common Burnet effective against various soil-borne plant pathogens, and may be useful to grow as antagonistic plants in mixed medicinal herb crops.

Garden Burnet can be grown as a cover crop in vineyards or around berry crops. It helps reduce soil erosion, good weed control, due to allelopathic properties and low growth during the summer. The seeds will germinate on infertile and dry sites, making it a good choice for reclamation work.

It can be grown from seed, or root divisions. Removing the flower heads will give more leaf growth.

The fruit contains two seeds that usually result in both germinating and then competing so that one dominates and the other dies.

Salad burnet lower flowers are male or hermaphrodite, the middle hermaphrodite and the upper female.

It grows best in pH 7-8.5 soil, well drained and sunny. It is not drought resistant but can survive on little water.

MEDICINAL

CONSTITUENTS- *S. officinalis* root- flavonoids including rutin and flavone sulphates, catechol type tannins (17%), gallic acid, triterpene glycosides including the aglycones pomolic acid (genin 19-alpha-hydroxyursolic acid), tormentosolic acid, tormentolic acid and saponins such as ziyuglycosides I and II, (sanguisorbin 2.5-4.0%), diyu glucosides, various phenolics including 4-O-beta-D-glucopyranosy-5-hydroxy-3-methoxybenzoate, 3,3',4'-tri-O-methylellagic acid, fisetinidol-(4alpha-8)-catechin, and (+)-catechin; carboxyl steroids including beta sitosterol; glucose, vitamin A, C, and volatile oils.

Sanguisorbin separates into sanguisorbigenin and valeric acid upon hydrolysis.

S. minor- 23-hydroxy-tormentic acid, and tormentic acid ester glucoside; hydroquinones, resorcinol, catechol, pyrogallol and gallic acid.

Both Common and Salad Burnet may be useful in the prevention and treatment of Alzheimer's disease.

Work by da Rocha MD et al, *CNS Neurolo Disord Drug Targets* 2011 10:2 251-70 found sixteen plants, including *S. officinalis* with potential to prevent amyloid plaque.

Salad Burnet was identified as the strongest acetylcholinesterase inhibitor in a study of Portuguese plants, and rated highly as an anti-oxidant agent. Ferreira et al, *J Ethnopharm* 2006 108 31-37.

Great Burnet is used for a number of female disorders, including menorrhagia during peri-menopause as well as hot flushes. The herb relieves diarrhea, dysentery, ulcerative colitis, enteritis, hemorrhoids, varicose veins, and phlebitis due in part to astringent, tonic, anti-bacterial, hemostatic and anti-hemorrhagic properties.

The herb can be poulticed and applied to external cuts and wounds.

The root is widely used in Traditional Chinese Medicine, and known as **DI YU, CHI YU, YU CHI,** or **SUAN ZHI**. This relates to the plant sprouts creeping along the ground, and the long leaves resembling elm.

Other names of interest are **HUNG TI YU**, translating as Red Bloodwort, and **HSUEH CHIEN TS'AO**, meaning Bloody Arrow Grass. In both Japan and Korea, the plant is known as **JIYU**.

The roots are bitter, sour, astringent, cool and dry, with the main activity affecting the liver and large intestine.

With a descending nature and ability to cool blood, clear heat and retain blood in body, it is considered one of our finest cooling astringent hemostatic herbs.

The compound 3, 3', 4-tri-O-methylellagic acid has been found responsible for controlling bleeding.

They are gathered in fall and dried for use in treating various hemostatic and anti-inflammatory conditions that require dispelling heat and tightening tissue. Peridontal gum disease would be one example of its use.

One study of 40 patients with bleeding after tooth extraction found topical application stopped bleeding in 3-5 minutes. *Chin Herb* 1988 469-73.

Other uses would include bleeding hemorrhoids, bloody stool, nosebleeds, menstrual or menopausal flooding or excessive bleeding, childbirth hemorrhage, and coughing up blood.

Extracts show anti-thrombin and anti-cancer activity. Goun EA et al, *J Ethnopharm* 2002 81 337-342.

For uterine bleeding, combine with cattail pollen, while for bleeding hemorrhoids add some goldthread. Also use as a retention douche for cervical erosion.

It is listed as 19th out of 250 potential anti-fertility plants in work by Duke & Ayensu, *Med Plants of China* 1985.

The root helps relieve vaginal discharge and women with milk stagnation pain, such as mastitis.

It appears to ease feelings of nausea and vomiting, by settling down the digestive tract. It helps ease infection and inflammation of the intestinal tract, and may be useful in ulcerative colitis.

A study of 91 patients with bacterial dysentery treated with a decoction three times daily showed 95.6% effectiveness. *Human J Med Herbology* 1978 3:18.

Difficult skin problems, including childhood eczema, respond well, due in part to the mild anti-bacterial and anti-fungal activity of the herb.

In laboratory studies, the charred and powdered root has been shown to decrease the amount of exudation from wounds, and helps to dry them up.

Rabbits exhibit much faster blood coagulation; and pigeons exhibit anti-emetic properties. Be careful with your pets!

Decoctions of the root completely inhibit pneumonia bacteria, and strongly inhibit *Pseudomonas aeruginosa, Bacillus typhi,* and *Shigella dysenteriae.*

Kim et al, *Phyto Res* 15:8 found the herb possesses anti-viral activity, specifically against hepatitis B.

Chen CuiPing et al, *Journal of Traditional Medicines* 2001 18:1 suggests root extracts help protect the kidneys from oxidative damage caused by drugs.

The herb appears to be of benefit in bronchial asthma due to hemeoxygenase up-regulation. Lee et al, *Int J Mol Med* 2010 26:2.

Work by Liao et al, *Evid Based Compl Alt Med* 2008 5:4 found the root one of the most anti-oxidant herbs tested at 1940 micromol TE/gram. The bitter, sour and cold attributes appear to be related to higher activity in general.

Yokozawa et al, *Bio Pharm Bulletin* 2000 23:6 found sanguiin H-6 the most active component of the root with respect to nitric oxide suppression. This follows work by Konishi in volume 2 of same year indicating sanquiin H-11 is a potent inhibitor of chemo-attractant-dependent and independent neutrophil movement. This suggests anti-inflammatory potential.

The root contains ziyu-glycosides and associated methyl esters that inhibit both tissue factor activity and tumor necrosis factor-alpha and may be useful in the inhibition of septic shock and atherosclerosis. Cho et al, *Planta Med* 2006 72.

Ziyuglycoside I has been identified as a good candidate for anti-wrinkle cosmetic formulations. Kim et al, *Biosci Biotech Biochem* 2008 72:2. It reduces the enzyme elastase which breaks down elastin and collagen and prevent wrinkle formation, in a study on volunteers for 12 weeks.

Work by Bastow et al, 1993 on H-6, a cytotoxic dimeric ellagitannin, showed inhibition of DNA topoisomerase.

Small doses appear to decrease intestinal spasms, while larger amounts aggravate.

It appears to be useful in bronchial asthma with an allergic origin due to HO-1 upregulation. Lee et al, *Int J Mol Med* 2010 26:2.

Mild hypotensive action was noted in rabbits. The root may be useful in the therapeutic treatment of strokes. Nguyen et al, *Biol Pharm Bull* 2008 31:11 found extracts inhibit H2O2 induced neuronal death by interfering with Ca2+, inhibition of glutamate release, and generation of reactive oxygen species.

Goun et al, looked at 45 plants native to Russia, and screened them for activity against cancer. Eight of the plants showed 90% inhibition of thrombin, and 9 showed 90% or higher inhibition leukemia L1210 cells; with *S. officinalis* showing high activity against both. *J Ethnopharm* 2002 81:3.

The herb induced apoptosis and inhibited angiogenesis in an *in vitro* trial on human breast cancer cell lines. Wang Z et al, *Expert Opin Ther Targets* 2012 March 16 Supplement 79-89.

Tinctures show cytotoxicity against PC3 prostate cancer cell lines. Choi et al, *Mol Med Report* 2012 6:3.

Both aerial parts and rhizome ethanol extracts show activity against various bacteria. Kokoska et al, *J Ethnopharm* 2002 82 51-3.

These include *Pseudomonas aeruginosa, Salmonella typhi, S. paratyphi, Proteus vulgaris, Staphylococcus aureus* and *Shigella dysenteriae.*

Garden Burnet (*S. minor magnolli*) has been shown to possess anti-viral activity.

Abad et al, *Phytotherapy Research* 2000 14:8 showed extracts at 50-125 micrograms per ml, effective against herpes simplex type (cold sores), and vesicular stomatitis virus. It also possesses anti-HIV activity *in vitro*. Bedoya et al, *J Ethnopharm* 2001 77 113-6.

Salad or Garden Burnet (*S. minor*) was investigated at University of Alberta by Sadari et al, and published in *Pharmaceutical Biology* 1998 36:3.

Crude extracts of the plant were found to possess anti-fungal activity against *Aspergillus, Candida* and *Cryptococcus*.

Both the root and aerial parts contain tormentic acid compounds that exhibit hypoglycemic properties.

Dried root decoctions help relieve diarrhea, including bloody type, associated with viral infections. The root tincture can be used as well in cool water.

This may be of value in respiratory conditions such as inflammation, infection and sore throats.

HOMEOPATHY

Sanguisorba is indicated for venous congestion and passive hemorrhages; for varicosities of the lower extremities, dysentery.

It is also used for cases of long lasting profuse menses with head congestion and painful limbs in sensitive, irritable patients. Climacteric hemorrhages.

Sanguisorba officinalis is used for profuse, long lasting menses, especially in nervous patients with congestive symptoms to head and limbs.

Patients communicate and share their suffering through blood, Holy Communion.

Stay with their suffering from loss of fluids, diarrhea, uterine bleedings, endure it as a way of life. The more I suffer the closer I am to God. See many doctors, associated with concept of suffering. This is the most syphilitic, self-destructive remedy of the Rosaceae.

DOSE- Second and third potency. Based on clinical from Boericke and observations by Mangialavori.

HYDROSOL

Great Burnet/Pimpernel water works with too cold a mother. It is combined with castoreum water for gout, and provokes the menses.

Small Burnet water is for stone and gravel, bladder and kidney problems, as well as a wash for hands and face. **BRUNSCHWIG**

FLOWER ESSENCES

Sitka Burnet (*S. stipulata*) flower essence is for healing the past on all levels; and helps us identify issues that are contributing to internal conflict. It works with individuals to bring forth the full potential for healing that lies within a given process. **ALASKA**

Salad Burnet (*P. sanguisorba*) essence overcomes depression from unfulfilled desires in relationships. When the romance fades, it's time to surrender to the nurturing this essence provides. As melancholy lifts, nutrient uptake and dispersion increases, enhancing blood volume and neuromuscular response. **PETITE FLEUR**

Greater Burnet (*S. officinalis*) essence is related to the qualities of love and affection. **MIRIANA**

PERSONALITY TRAITS

Most Rosaceae were used to prevent bleeding, such as Sanguisorba from Latin, sanguis, blood, and sorbeo, to absorb. Christian iconography suggests that the giving of blood is a kind of sacrifice. By sacrificing, by giving sacrum is to make something holy. The pain of sacrifice is to not know who you are. **MANGIALAVORI**

ASTROLOGY

In the burnet, even more than in the agrimony and meadowsweet, the individual flowers do not stretch out so far. They form tightly crowded, round flower heads, which are elevated above the vegetative region by means of long internodes. In the midsummer meadows, we often see the brownish-red heads of the greater burnet standing above the other plants. The tiny flowers turn in all directions. There are but few plants in which the flowering process turns towards the atmosphere so perfectly. These flower heads are like a higher stage of the flowering process.

In strange combination with a strong inhibition or contraction into one center, this turning to the surrounding space escalates in the burnet as the expression of Saturn in the region of the flower. **KRANICH**

RECIPES

TINCTURE- 2-5 ml three times daily. Plant tinctures are prepared from the whole plant including root, 1:5 and 40% with dry material and 1:2 and 50% with fresh plant. The dry tincture is better for hemostatic activity.

DECOCTION- 8-15 grams. The sliced root is dry fried until blackened to decrease its cold nature and reduce bleeding.

CAUTION- Do not use *S. officinalis* in cold or weak conditions, especially a deficiency of Chi causing uterine bleeding. It is used to reduce hot, damp conditions.

Sanguisorba is contraindicated both orally and locally for those suffering hepatitis, and should not be used topically to treat large area burns.

It may interact with ciprofloxacin and concurrent use is to be avoided.

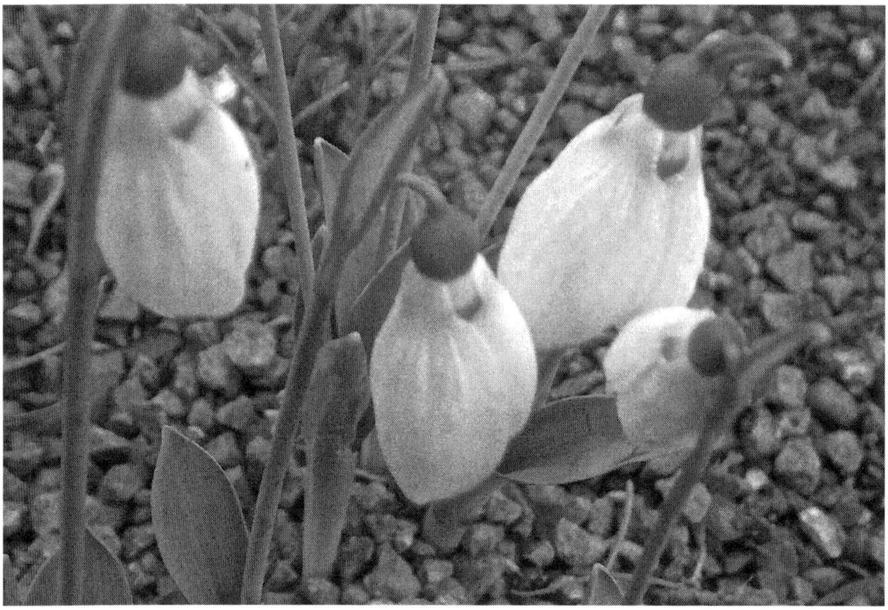

Snowdrops

SNOWDROP
(*Galanthus nivalis* L.)
PARTS USED- bulbs

And the snowdrop, wakened by his song,

Peeps tremblingly forth,

From her bed of cold still slumber,

To gaze upon the earth. **TWAMLEY**

Galanthus is from the Greek **GALA** meaning white or milk and **ANTHOS** meaning flower. Nivalis means growing near snow. In France it is known as *Perce Neige*.

Snowdrop came into Elizabethan English as a direct translation from the German **SCHNEETROPFEN**, meaning snow droplet, after a style of pendulant earring popular in the 16th century.

Snowdrop is a welcome spring flower that is hardy enough for prairie gardens. There are a multitude of cultivars available, but most are white flowered with green lips or markings at the tip.

The plant is small, only six inches or so, but in the right location, and with quantity, it can really look fine. The flowers have a mossy scent.

Snowdrops were said to have appeared as Adam and Eve were driven from the Garden of Eden. An angel consoled them through the cold, snowy, dark winter, and blew on a falling snowflake that touched the ground as a plant, giving hope.

The common Snowdrop was probably the antidote used by Odysseus to counter the effects of Circe's poisonous drugs in Homer's epic poem, The Odyssey. It was known as Moly as in HOLY MOLY.

If true, this is the first recorded use of galanthamine to reverse central anti-cholinergic intoxication. See below.

It was traditionally known as the Fair Maid of February, and their blooming was considered a sign of good luck for the coming year.

This is connected to the old custom of celebrating the Feast of Purification of St. Mary on February 2nd. At this feast, on Candlemas, young maidens would gather bunches of the snowdrops and wear them as symbols of purity. The flowers symbolize hope, and have been assigned this birth date. It was said, however, that bringing the flower indoors was unlucky if someone in the household was ill.

A few blossoms were sent by mail to warn off a man who expressed intentions.

An old Moldavian legend resembles Snow White by the Brothers Grimm, in the battle between the Winter Witch and the beautiful Lady Spring. Her name was Snowdrop.

Traditionally the mashed bulb was used as a poultice for frostbite injury.

Grieve says that an old manuscript of 1465, called the plant, *Leucis i viola alba*, and classified it as an emmenagogue. "Placed under narcissi, its healing properties are stated to be 'digestive, resolutive and consolidante'."

It has been used in Eastern Europe, as a preparation called Nivalin, for a wide variety of nerve tissue degeneration conditions including poliomyelitis, Alzheimer's disease, muscular dystrophy and myasthenia gravis.

A recent paper in The Lancet, found snowdrop lectins bind strongly to human white blood cell protein.

The experiments were carried out directly on humans who were fed the lectin in Dundee, Scotland. Researchers found that white blood cells, but not red cells, have many proteins that bound strongly to the lectin. The implications for the use of snowdrop in GM foods are obvious.

Giant Snowdrop (*G. elwesii*) grows well on the West Coast, but is not hardy enough for the prairie winters. All Snowdrop bulbs should be lifted and divided immediately after flowering in harsher climates.

MEDICINAL

CONSTITUENTS- bulb- galanthamine, hippeastrine, lycorine, narvedine, tazettine, nivalidine, narwedine, ungeremine, hamayne, ismine.

Galanthamine is a watcr-soluble alkaloid from snowdrop root and daffodils above.

It is a selective, competitive acetyl-cholinesterase inhibitor that is reversible with time. Individuals with Alzheimer's disease are deficient in the neurotransmitter acetylcholine.

It inhibits erythrocyte acetylcholinase better than brain acetylcholinase; is nearly 100% bio-available and crosses the blood-brain barrier.

It antagonizes muscle relaxation caused by non-depolarizing, curare-like muscle relaxants; and is used post-operatively to reverse the effects of neuromuscular blockers. In other words, galanthamine is strongly analgesic. Schuh et al, *Anaesthesist* 1976 25:9.

In one study of healthy male volunteers, galanthamine reversed central anti-cholinergic syndrome induced by scopolamine. Baraka & Harik, *JAMA* 1977.

Preliminary clinical trials with synthetic galanthamine with Alzheimer's disease have provided mixed results. Dal-Bianco et al, *J Neural Transmission Supplementum* 1991 33.

In one placebo-controlled study by Kewitz et al, *Neuropsychopharmacology* 1994 10, of 95 patients with mild to moderate Alzheimer's disease, clinical evaluation indicates considerably less deterioration in patients after ten weeks of treatment.

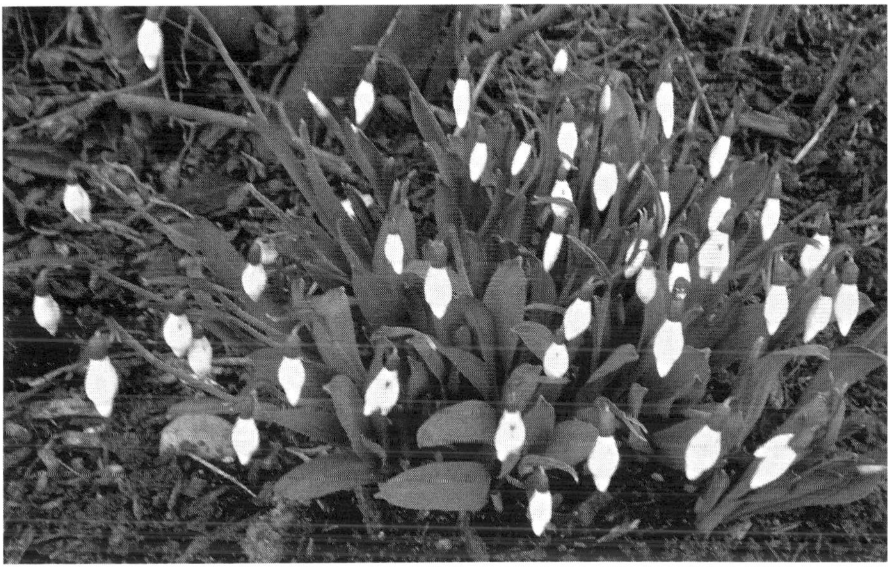

Snowdrops

And in the *Journal of Pharmacology and Experimental Therapeutics* 1996 227, Bores et al, found acetylcholinesterase inhibitors, including galanthamine useful in Alzheimer's disease.

In addition to being a cholinesterase inhibitor, galanthamine is a non-competitive nicotinic channel activator, which may also be of value in the disease.

According to Frans Vermeulen "the long-term efficacy of galanthamine is attributed to its unique dual mechanism of action. Like other Alzheimer's disease treatments, the substance enhances levels of the neurotransmitter acetylcholine and additionally, unlike the others, it has a modulating effect on the brain's nicotinic receptors, increasing their effectiveness."

It is interesting to note that the risk of developing Alzheimer's disease is halved in tobacco smokers. Lee, *Neuroepidemiology* 1994 13. This is because nicotine mimics the effect of acetylcholine.

The use of galanthamine as a synthetic drug, is approved in Austria. Common trade names include Jilkon, Lycoremin, and Nivalin.

Work by Snorrason in Iceland treated 49 chronic fatigue patients with galanthamine. Thirty-nine patients completed the trial, and 43% reported 50% improvement in fatigue, myalgia and sleep and 70% reported 30% improvement, compared to only 10% in placebo group. Snorrason et al, *J Chronic Fatigue Syndrome* 1996 2:2-3 35-54.

In the fall of 2001, Health Canada approved the drug Reminyl (galanthamine hydrobromide) for mild to moderate Alzheimer's and related dementia.

Narwedine, a constituent from bulb, was identified by Harborne and Baxter in 1993. It has been found effective in lowering blood pressure, decreasing cardiac contraction frequency and yet raising amplitude, increasing both respiration amplitude and frequency and potentiating the effect of morphine.

Lycorine produces significant sedative activity in lab studies, and increases the analgesic effects of corydalis.

At one time, Snowdrop extracts were being investigated for use in glaucoma.

Extracts of Giant Snowdrop (*G. elwesii*) have been shown to exhibit potent anti-herpes simplex virus activity. Hudson et al, *Pharm Bio* 2000 38:3.

Galanthus species have been found to exhibit cytotoxic activity against cervical, colon and acute myeloid leukemia human cell lines. Jokhadze et al, *Phyto Res* 2007 21:7.

For frostbite or chilblains, make a poultice of the crushed bulbs and apply to the affected area.

Snowdrop extracts significantly reduced salmonella numbers in infected mice. Naughton et al, *J Appl Microbiol* 2000 88:4.

It inhibited the growth of *Chlamydia trachomatis* by binding to a glycoprotein in the organism. Amim et al, *APMIS* 1995 103:10.

Gilljam et al, *AIDS Res Hum Retroviruses* 1993 9:5 found a strong immune response when the glyco-proteins of HIV-1, HIV-2 and SIV were purified with snowdrop extract.

Galanthamine may be used as an antidote to atropine poisoning and is antagonist to morphine and other narcotics.

The Red Spider Lily (*Lycoris radiata*) contains lycorine and galanthamine; but the beautiful plant is hardy only to zones 6-7.

An excellent review of Snowdrop and galanthamine is Heinrich et al, *Journal of Ethnopharmacology* 2004 92 147-62.

HOMEOPATHY

Snowdrop (*G. nivalis*) is indicated for faintness, and sinking sensations. There is a sore, dry throat with dull headache. The patient is half conscious and worried feeling during sleep. The heart is weak with sensation of collapse as if they must fall. Pulse very irregular, rapid and uneven, violent palpitations.

Systolic murmur at apex. Therapeutically, a decided benefit in cases of Mitral Regurgitation, with broken down compensation. Myocarditis, with some degree of mitral insufficiency.

DOSE- First to 5th potency. The proving was by Dr. A Whiting of Vancouver, BC.

A meditative proving by Madeline Evans in England added fear of change, enormous anxiety and stammering, desire to hide, great need of company.

It helps clear deep shock and trauma, nervous complaints, unrest and hunger. Vision is affected, with inability to fix the eyes. It appears to lower blood pressure very quickly in acute situations.

Three case studies in *Plants* Volume One by Vermeulen and Johnston pages 151-154.

FLOWER ESSENCES

Snowdrop (*G. nivalis*) flower essence helps combine enthusiasm, inspiration and joyful exploration of life experiences. It embodies the qualities of personal power and leadership. It is the flower essence for letting go, having fun and lightening up.

It helps dissolve energy blockages and personal holding patterns which prevent energy from moving freely in the body.

Physically it impacts on disorders where freedom of physical expression is paralyzed or distorted in some manner, such as arthritis, multiple sclerosis, poliomyelitis, or cerebral palsy. It strengthens the will and dissolves paralyzing fear, and helps us get mobilized.

PACIFIC

Single Snowdrop (*G. nivalis*) is the flower remedy for those experiencing difficulties in breaking through to new levels of awareness and consciousness. This remedy is particularly for those where these is vulnerability to corruption, this leading to a falling back into the old patterns which they are trying to leave behind. At the back of this vulnerability is the fear of letting go of comfortable old identities and facing an apparently bleaker world. **BAILEY**

Double Snowdrop (*G. nivalis* x flore-pena) is for those who need to have more flexibility, who have become frozen in their attitudes… They need the insight to see that everything is constantly changing and that change, however uncomfortable it may feel at times, is a fact of life. It is fear of change that is the main Double Snowdrop characteristic. **BAILEY**

Snowdrop (*G. nivalis*) flower essence allows us to surrender to the end of past events and attachments in life. In the death of the old we find the seed of our eternal inner light and–behold new vistas; immortality. It is indicating in personal darkness and suffering, negative or destructive attitudes, and the fear of death and dying. It is usefu for the depression related to SAD, or seasonal affective disorder, and for the dark night of the soul. The essence of Snowdrop allows us to access deep inner stillness and to surrender to the processes whereby we can release the past. **FINDHORN**

Snowdrop flower essence is for the release of deep pain, tears and old traumas that have been stuck for a long time. Especially when these originate from the handing-in of the heart and you did not stand by yourself and your feelings. When you have done everything for the other and have forgotten yourself. When you do everything the other says, while you know that it should be done differently. To find your own beauty and importance again. To do things you like to do, to feel free. The essence brings a stronger trust, deep down in the base. Joyful refreshing energy after the dark emotional winter. **BLOESEM**

As a flower essence, Snowdrop works on the throat, heart and solar plexus chakra- allowing energy to run unhindered with force from the universe. It creates a surge of energy in the chest to give the momentum to move forward from "issues". It can be taken when you're feeling frustrated or just worn down. **OLIVE**

SPIRITUAL PROPERTIES

When Adam and Eve were turned from the Garden of Eden, it was a cold winter day. They quickly had to find shelter in a cave, learn to find food, and make clothing from animal skins.

But Eve missed the flowers most of all. One snowy day, Eve crept back towards the Garden, hoping for a glimpse of green. But however she approached, a guardian angel would prevent her getting close.

She finally gave up and turned towards home, weeping. The guardian angel saw her pain, and stepping away from the gates held out his hand and caught one of the falling snowflakes. He then raised his hand and gently blew until it turned into a beautiful snowdrop flower.

He presented it to Eve saying, "Let this bloom be a reminder that winter will not last forever". **FERGUSON**

PERSONALITY TRAITS

In the 19th century, Hans Christian Andersen wrote a tale titled, The Snowdrop. The story vividly tells how excited Sunbeams welcomed the snowdrop and said:

"Beautiful Flower! How graceful and delicate you are! You are the first, you are the only one! You are the bell that rings out for summer, beautiful summer, over country and town."

However, the Wind and Weather said, "You have come too early. We have still the power, and you shall feel it, and give it up to us. You should have stayed quietly at home and not have run out to make a display of yourself. Your time is not come yet!"

But the flower had more strength than she herself knew. She was strong in joy and faith in the summer, which would be sure to come, which had been announced by her deep longing and confirmed by the warm sunlight; and so she remained standing in confidence in the snow in her white garment, bending her head even while the snowflakes fell thick and heavy, and the icy winds swept over her.

The story then compares the snowdrop to a certain poet who came too early, before his time, and therefore he had to taste the sharp winds. And so it is for others who dare to step out ahead of the crowd, who despite having to face biting criticism, confidently chime their bells of hope. Like the little snowdrop, they too can triumph.

G. MOHAMMED

If you listen closely enough you can almost hear the quiet groaning of the leafy earth as the spears of snowdrops split it apart, thrusting their grey-green shoots every upwards…At first one or two shoots peer outwards, inspecting the wintry scene like animals emerging gingerly from hibernation, sniffing the air. **CAROL KLEIN**

RECIPES

TABLETS- Galanthamine- Initially, 5 mg three times daily, increasing to 30-40 mg daily. Dosage should reduce acetyl-cholinesterase activity by 35-60%.

IV- 0.3 mg/kg for reversal of neuromuscular blockers.

CAUTION- Do not use with MAO inhibitors, and it is of course, contraindicated in Parkinson's disease and epilepsy.

Organophosphate fertilizers that inhibit acetyl-cholinesterase and galanthamine should not be used together. In fact, fertilizers with this effect should be avoided by anyone who cares about their health.

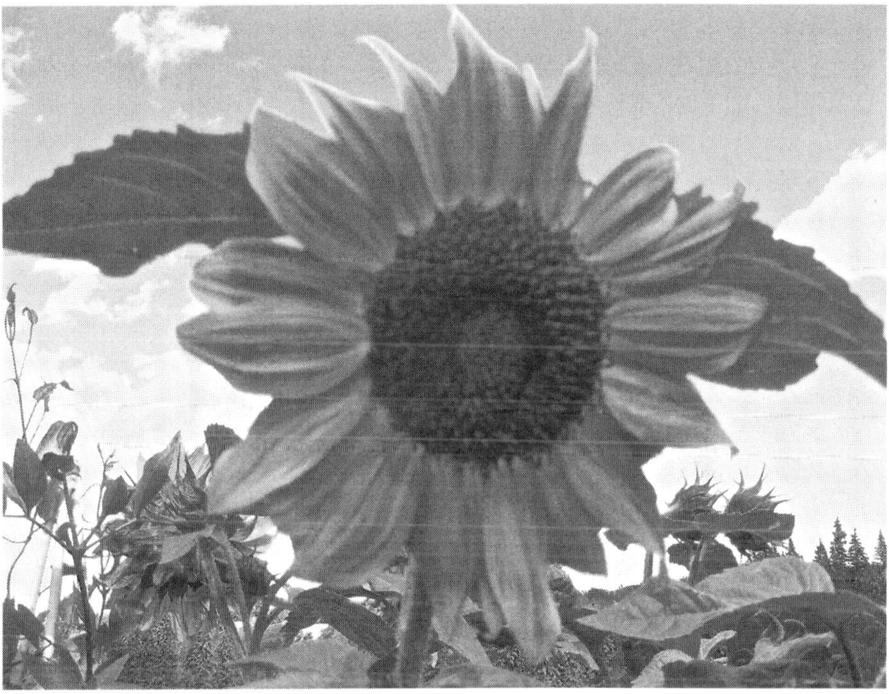

Sunflower

SUNFLOWER
(*Helianthus annuus* L.)
(*H. annuus ssp. lenticularis*)
PRAIRIE SUNFLOWER
(*H. couplandii* Boivin.)
(*H. aridus*)
(*H. petiolaris*)
BEAUTIFUL SUNFLOWER
RHOMBIC LVD SUNFLOWER
(*H. rigidus*)
(*H. subrhomboideus*)
(*H. laetiflorus*)
(*H. pauciflorus* Nutt.)
(*H. pauciflorus* ssp. *subrhomboideus*)
NARROW-LEAVED SUNFLOWER
(*H. maximiliani* Schrad.)

NUTTALL'S SUNFLOWER
COMMON TALL SUNFLOWER
(***H. nuttallii*** Torr. & Gray)
JERUSALEM ARTICHOKE
(***H. tuberosus*** L.)
FUSEAU J. ARTICHOKE
(***H. tuberosus*** L.)
PARTS USED- seed, flower, stem, pith, root

My summer home is the fairest of all, with a morning glory roof and sunflower walls! **LOVEJOY**

The full Sunflower blew
And became a starre of Bartholomew.
We're not our skin of grime... we're all beautiful golden sunflowers inside. **ALLEN GINSBERG**

Ah, sunflower! weary of time
Who countest the steps of the sun
Seeking after that sweet golden clime
Where the traveler's journey is done. **WILLIAM BLAKE**

These petals (sunflower) are an uncompromising yellow-orange. The color seems to contain all the energy this planet will ever need. This color could power a nuclear reactor. It rings like a carillon. It hits me, with a little punch, in the solar plexus. **RUSSELL**

Helianthus is from the Latin **HELIO** for Sun, and **ANTHOS**, meaning flower. Helios was the Greek god of the sun, who was drowned by his uncles, the Titans, and then raised to the sky. Heliotropism, or following the sun, is related term. Rigidus means rigid, and subrhomboideus refers to the diamond-shaped leaves.

Annuus means annual, tuberosus suggests tubers. Prince Maximilian Alexander Philipp of Wied-Neuwied, was a major general in the Prussian army, who later devoted himself to natural history and ethnology.

He traveled Brazil in the early 1800s and in 1832 explored North America, spending the winter in Fort Clark, now Bismarck, North Dakota. Accompanying him was Karl Bodmer, who painted landscapes and portraits of the Plains tribes.

Girasole means Sunflower in Italian, from **GIRARE**, meaning to turn around, and **SOLE**, the sun; and is thought the origin of Jerusalem. Others believe that Girasol was term originally used for the fire opal and castor bean long before it was attached to the Sunflower. One suggestion is that Petrus Hondius planted a small tuber in Ter Neusens, Holland and it distributed from there in 1618. They were called Artichoke Apples of Ter-Neusen, and when they arrived in England somehow became converted to Jerusalem.

Artichoke is so named for its similar texture to Globe Artichoke heart. In Italy, ironically, it is called *Girasole di Canada*. Fuseau is from the French, referring to the distinctive spindle shape of the tubers. The uniform shape may provide greater marketing opportunities.

The Sunflower is associated with fire and the sun; and of course, masculine energy.

It grows quickly taking full advantage the 1,300,000,000,000,000,000, 000,000 calories of energy striking the earth each year. Or, put another way, 4.3 pounds of sunlight hit the earth every second.

It was once believed that the truth in any matter is revealed by sleeping with a sunflower under the bed. If you cut a sunflower at sunset while making a wish, it will come true before the next sunset.

To dream of sunflowers means your pride will be wounded, but to grow them in your garden is good luck.

The sunflower is believed native to the southwestern United States. In Mexico, the plant known as **CHIMAIATI**, was cultivated nearly 4600 years ago, according to new research.

It is sometimes known as Maiz de Tejas, suggesting it was introduced from the north in exchange for squash, beans and corn. This is uncertain.

The Aztecs have replicated the design of sunflower in body jewelry for the same three millennium. The Mayans made an extract of the petals, which they drank as an aphrodisiac. This may be due, in part to the chlorogenic acid, which has sexually stimulating effects.

Lonicerus suggested cooking the fresh petals in oil and eating them to give "great power to marital works".

Although native to the Americas, it was immediately valued when introduced to Europe. In Holland, the plant is used for marsh reclamation. Russia is the largest producer of sunflowers in the world, due in part to the Russian Orthodox Church, that forbade most oil-containing foods during Lent or forty days before Christmas.

The radiant petals came to symbolize the sun and usurped the flower language of heliotrope, as a symbol of devotion.

Oscar Wilde took on the flower as his personal symbol and emblem of the Aesthetic Movement. This was a reaction to the industrial age and found the flower's image carved into chair backs, glazed on vases and on iron railings.

Sunflower is the floral emblem of both Russia and Peru, where I spent a few years studying plant medicines and the state flower of Kansas. Only the unopened flower buds track the sun back and forth.

Ironically, an adjoining state, has declared it a noxious weed. It makes a good companion plant with calendula, or angelica.

In ancient Peru, the Maidens of the Sun who were the virgins of the Inca, wore large gold suns to cover their breasts. This is viewed by some authors, as a representation of sunflowers, but there is no evidence it was cultivated in Peru or any part of South America until recent times.

The juice, expressed from the fresh stems, was used for anointing oneself if they wished to be virtuous.

The Cree of Alberta call the Wild Sunflower, **PISIMONEPEHKAN**.

They, and many others, used the native sunflower for its seeds. They were dried over a fire, and ground lightly to remove the shells, and then ground into a meal or flour for making porridge by boiling, or flat breads in grease, or bone marrow.

The small, flat sunflower cakes were often carried as a lightweight and high energy food source.

Seeds from about 2850 years ago were approximately one half the length of present day seeds.

The seeds were boiled for oil that was rubbed on the body and used to groom hair. The leaves have been used for treating kidney problems.

The Omaha Ponca call the plant **ZHA ZI** meaning yellow weed. The Teton Dakota boiled the sunflower heads, without bracts, as a remedy for pulmonary disease and chest pain.

The Pawnee pounded the seeds together with unidentified roots, and taken in a dry form by a woman who becomes pregnant while still nursing a child. This was done in order that the nursing baby would not become sick.

Samuel de Champlain observed cultivated sunflowers in eastern Canada as early as 1615.

The Ojibwa crushed thc root and applied it as a wet dressing to draw blisters. Some Plains tribes mixed the ground seed with buffalo bone marrow to make a type of firm pudding. The Cochiti smeared the sticky juice of fresh stems on wounds to prevent infection.

The Navajo used the sunflower for prenatal problems believed caused by an eclipse of the sun. The Hopi cultivated a purple seed Sunflower that was boiled for dyeing textiles and baskets.

In Mexico, the leaves and stems are tinctured to treat arthritis and sore muscles externally, whilc an infusion is given to relieve catarrh, and fevers. The dry or green leaves are decocted and the liquid added to baths for rheumatism or pain in the bones.

The flowers and seeds can be juiced and taken on an empty stomach for intermittent fevers, edema, cancer, palsy, and is considered a specific for bladder and kidney stones.

While traveling in Venezuela, I often found the leaves and flowers sold separately by street herbalists. The flowers are decocted for heart weakness, while leaf poultices are applied to the abdomen in cases of distress or to relieve rheumatic pain.

Sunflower is an annual grown commercially on about 150,000 acres across the three prairie provinces, mainly for the birdseed and confectionary market.

The tallest sunflower recorded in Guinness World Records, grown in 1986, was 7.7 metres tall. At peak of growth, they can grow up to 30 cm a day. The record for most heads is 129, produced in Michigan in 2000. The shortest bonsai mature sunflower was just over five cm. The record diameter sunflower head was grown in Maple Ridge, BC and measured 82 cm.

Sunflower is a familiar Prairie crop, more widely grown in Saskatchewan and Manitoba than in Alberta.

In 1999, Saskatchewan farmers seeded 65000 acres, and produced 78 million pounds of seed. This was up significantly from 1998, when only 40000 acres were seeded. Farmers in Manitoba harvested 145000 acres in 2000, accounting for 85% of the total Western Canada production.

Manitoba and Saskatchewan are the primary producers, with any sunflowers for vegetable oil contracted to US companies. A plant in Altona, Manitoba closed its doors in 1996. Yields of about one ton of seed per acre can be expected on average, and worth about $300.

The larger seed is used for the confection market and is 20/64th of an inch or larger (known as the 20s in the industry). This can bring 23 to 24 cents a pound, with average yield of 2000 pounds per acre. The hull accounts for 46% of the weight of in shell product. The kernel is 47% fat, 23% protein, and 18% carbohydrate.

New hybrids, collectively called NuSun, produce sunflower oil that is several times higher in oleic acid than traditional sunflower oil. It is estimated that by the year 2001, the United States acreage of oilseed sunflowers could double from the present 2.2 million, due to increased demand. North Dakota planted 1.7 million acres in 2000.

Bees help pollination and produce a sunflower honey much in demand.

Sunflower milk, long popular in the Far East and Japan, is manufactured similar to the process for soymilk production.

Sunflower seed butter is slightly greener and more plastic than peanut butter, but shows good nutritional value.

The seeds can be roasted and ground as a coffee substitute, or sprouted for their edible, tasty green that takes approximately ten days to fully mature. Use the black oil sprouting variety, as 99% of the shells fall off naturally.

In Turkey and Persia, a tincture is prepared from the seeds with wine as a substitute for quinine in intermittent fevers. In China, the seeds are used to treat dysentery, in Brazil the leaves are infused for asthma, and in Cuba, a decoction of flowers is used for the common cold.

The unopened flower buds can be steamed and eaten like artichokes.

A sunflour was produced and marketed many years ago. It had to be mixed with wheat flour because of the high oil content, but made superior bakery goods.

Gonzalez-Perez et al at Wageningen University, The Netherlands, found a method suitable for producing sunflower seed protein isolate free of chlorogenic acid which reduces digestibility, functionality and a dark colour. *J Agric Food Chem* 2002 50.

Three years later, the same authors in same journal, reported on the formation and stability of foams from sunflower protein. The work continues.

Soapstock is produced when hexane and other chemicals are used to extract and refine edible oil from sunflower and safflower seeds. It is presently added to animal feed, but could have new uses.

First, researchers had to rid soapstock of its water and hexane, without eliminating desirable properties. Then they spread the soapstock paste onto glass plates and spheres to form thin, flexible films.

This gummy, amber coloured byproduct could become a new biodegradable film for encapsulating fungicides and slow release chemicals, and packaging fresh produce, such as bell peppers. They are testing soapstock gel for hair styling and colouring.

Sunflower seed protein has visco-elastic properties that lend themselves to biodegradable product production.

The inflorescences of cultivated sunflowers contain a highly active anti-feedant for western corn root worms. Germacranolide angelates exhibit structural features similar to picrotoxinin, a gamma amino butyric acid (GABA) gated chloride channel antagonist. Two diterpenoid acids, 16-kauren-19-oic acid and trachyloban-19-oic acid, have been isolated from the florets of *H. annuus*. They have been shown to inhibit the growth of the sunflower moth, and other insects.

Virgin female sunflower moths, when exposed to the odour of pollen, begin signaling for males more intensely.

Sunflowers have been observed to accumulate scopoletin and ayapin around wound tissue. These compounds show strong fungicide and insecticide activity.

Somaclonal variants of sunflower containing elevated levels of ayapin have shown improved anti-feeding resistance.

The leaves, if carefully dried, can be used as a substitute for tobacco in cigar making; the flavour is said to greatly resemble that of mild Spanish tobacco.

Work by Macias et al, reported in the 1999 *Journal of Natural Products*, found heliannuals isolated from sunflower leaves have phytotoxic activity and potential as a natural herbicide.

Work by Harris et al, at Oregon State University looked at the feeding habits of rabbits on 14 different fresh greens. Out of 100 grams offered, the rabbits ate 98.4% of sunflower leaves, followed by red clover, carrot tops, cauliflower leaves (all 90+%), dandelion (83%), white clover (80%), Swiss chard (78%), corn leaves (66%), and amaranthus (65%).

Sunflower leaves contain fumaric acid, which substitutes for tartaric acid in beverages and baked products.

The leaves and stalks are infused in vodka in Russia for gout.

The left over stem fibre and seedless heads can be used for paper. The Chinese have used the fibre to make thread and weave into silk fabrics; while the Russians have made them into lightweight acoustic ceiling tile. Recent research by Marechal et al, in *Industrial Crops and Products*, 1999 10 shows that sunflower fibre is suitable for cardboard fibre.

The pith of the stem was used at one time for life preservers in Russia, having a greater buoyancy than either cork or reindeer's hair, and specific gravity of 0.028. The pith is like polystyrene and could find application in packaging and packing materials.

This pith is used as a mounting medium for microscope study.

They make great kindling for starting fires. They contain high amounts of phosphorus and potassium and can also be returned to the soil as fertilizer.

Sunflower meal contains 9.7% of di- and oligosaccharides, mainly sucrose, trehalose, and raffinose.

Arabinans and arabinogalactans are 9% and 13% respectively in the flour and protein concentrate.

Scientists at North Dakota State University have extracted various anthocyanins from sunflower hulls that have potential as red food colorants.

The hulls were at one time discarded or used for poultry litter. They can be used to produce blotting paper, and fibreboard.

Co-op Vegetable Oils, a Canadian firm, press the hulls into logs which are superior to coal for some purposes in cook stoves and furnaces.

Today, in Russia, the hulls are used to manufacture ethyl alcohol and furfural, in lining plywood, and in growing yeast. Nitrated or oxidated hulls are a rich source of organic nitrogen fertilizer. Efanov et al, *Chem Nat Comp* 2002 38:6, indicate sunflower hulls then stimulate pea growth.

The hulls may be useful in the removal of color dyes from dilute industrial effluent. Thinkaran et al, *J Hazard Mater* 2008 151:2-3. The petals yield a yellow dye.

The white central pith of the stalk contains nitre, which has been used in the past as a diuretic. It can be gathered like the white fuzz of mugwort as a form of moxa, something practiced by the Portuguese.

Flower infusions and decoctions are used as fly killers. Water extracts of the flowers have been shown to kill mice, but not rabbits in a most important laboratory experiment!

A University of Alberta professor and bio-organic chemist has recently received a grant to see if sunflowers stems can be bio-engineered to produce natural rubber. John Vederas hopes that by inserting genes from the Brazilian rubber tree into sunflowers he can increase the latex production of the stems from around 50 pounds per acre to around 800 pounds.

“At $1 US a pound, that’s a fairly high-valued crop”, he says. The southwestern Guayule bush may also be a source of genetic material for the project. The United States demand alone for rubber-derived finished goods is $28 billion annually.

Sunflowers help remediate areas of chemical and radiation pollution.

Near Chernobyl, in the Ukraine, where a nuclear reactor had a meltdown many years ago, sunflowers were grown on floating rafts in ponds full of cesium, and strontium. The plants flourished and absorbed 90% of the radioactivity from the water in the first generation. These radioactive minerals are then concentrated thousands of times greater than the surrounding water.

At the same time, be careful with cadmium rich soils. Sunflowers tend to accumulate the heavy metal in the seeds, at levels exceeding health standards. In one experiment conducted in Germany, the seeds were found to contain 1.1 mg/kg, even when the soil cadmium level was below the 3mg/kg widely accepted for agricultural use.

Sunflowers extract heavy metals such as lead, uranium, strontium, cesium, chromium, copper, manganese, nickel and zinc. They also show promise in degrading PAHs in soil.

Sunflower also uses a lot of carbon dioxide, each plant requiring 14 ounces per month. Industries requiring carbon credits need look no further.

Sunflower seeds, de-hulled, are used in veterinary medicine for horses suffering respiratory distress, coughs, and heaving of flanks.

In one study, researchers found that feeding dairy cows on kilogram of whole sunflower seed daily, increased milk yields substantially with little or no loss of protein or milk fat, and revenue increase of $2 per cow per day.

The sunflower grows in spirals of 21, 34, 55, 89 and 144 seeds, each number the sum of the previous two numbers. This pattern is found everywhere in nature, from pine needles, mullusc shells, parrot beaks and spiral galaxies. It is related to the golden mean, a basis for Egyptian pyramids and the Greek Parthenon, as well as art and music.

Even in our own ear's spiral shaped cochlea, musical notes vibrate to this same ratio. See Yarrow (Cardiovascular) for more information on Fabonacci numbers and golden mean.

Sunflower buds tend to follow the sun, but once opened, tend to face east, possibly to protect them on very hot days. This heliotropic movement called nutation results from the stems bending toward the sun. Growth is equalized at night, the stem slowly straightening out and at dawn again face east.

On cloudy days they remain facing east. The leaves are heliotropic and if removed the sunflower's head no longer follows the sun. Once the ray flowers are fully developed, movement ceases.

Bears and other animals feed on the tuberous roots of Nuttall's Sunflower, a perennial very closely related to Jerusalem Artichoke. The Cree call this particular Sunflower species, **OWTIYHIYMESKIYHKIY**, or sometimes **MITIYHIYMESKIYHKIY**.

The Cree of Alberta would use the mature root decoction to treat heart problems. The Navaho made an infusion of the dry crushed leaves for stomach troubles.

The leaves of *H. maximiliani* contain 8-beta-sarracinoyloxycumambranolide, which deters the feeding of the sunflower moth larvae. Various sesquiterpene lactones and diterpenes in all species are rich in anti-feedant and insecticidal potential.

Prairie Sunflower (*H. petiolaris*) was used, by Hopi as a "spider medicine". The Navaho used cold infusions of the flowers sprinkled on clothing for good luck in hunting. In British Columbia, the Thompsons powdered the leaves either alone or in an ointment for sores and swellings.

A tincture of the seeds can be used to treat sub-acute lung infections, as well as allergy related coughs. The tincture is also slightly diuretic.

When I lived near Joussard in the early 1970s, my mentor Jean Chancelet introduced me to Jerusalem Artichokes.

They are neither from Jerusalem nor Artichokes.

It was early spring, the ground still frozen, and the snow barely gone. I took a shovel and started digging where directed, and out popped these numerous tubers.

We cleaned and steamed them later that day, and the rest I took home to plant. By fall, they had reached ten feet, with small sunflower like faces.

The tubers have a crisp texture like water chestnuts, and a slightly coconut flavour.

They can be baked, boiled, roasted, or eaten raw, but in large quantities will cause gas and bloating.

The unopened buds of all these plants can be steamed and eaten like globe artichokes. The French explorer, Champlain, wrote that the roots tasted like artichokes, explaining half the name.

Various native tribes ate the roots. The Chippewa called them raw thing or **A'SKIBWAN'**. Champlain reported seeing them under cultivation near Cape Cod in 1605. The Cree name for the root was **ASKIPAW**, which was corrupted by Europeans into Esquebois. This is very similar to the Cree name for potato, **ASKIPWAW**.

The Cheyenne name is **HOHINON**, and the Pawnee name is **KISU-SIT**, meaning long or tapering.

When introduced into England, it became known as Potato of Canada. The juice squeezed from the plant blossoms was formerly used to restore hair growth.

In the United States, both the tubers and above ground parts are used for livestock feed. The leaves contain a protein isolate rich in lysine, and an amino acid profile comparable to major cereal proteins.

Potential protein yield, from three monthly cuttings, is estimated to be 800 kg/hectare.

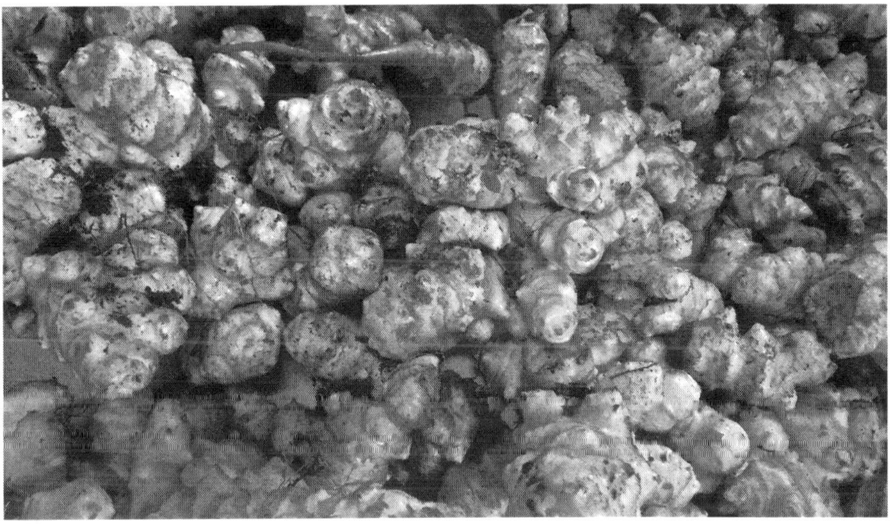

Fresh Jerusalem Artichoke tubers

In studies by Rawate and Hill at the University of Minnesota in 1985, a protein isolate obtained by water extraction from the tops contained 67-76% protein, also rich in lysine.

The tubers are rich in protein, with methionine the limiting amino acid, containing 58% of that found in eggs.

The tuber can be used in the manufacture of syrup, containing 70-80% fructose, and 20-30% glucose.

The tubers can be sliced and roasted in an oven as a coffee substitute. Combined with the roasted sunflower seed, you have a healthy, sweet beverage from two members of the same genus.

Methods to give high extraction rates of inulin (21%) from the dried tubers has been achieved.

Inulin demand as a prebiotic is increasing worldwide. A new Inulin plant, Asia's largest, has recently been completed in China. The first crop of 50,000 tonnes of tubers was expected to produce some 4500 tonnes of inulin in 2005.

Inulinase is present in inactive form, except during the germination period, one at pH 3, and the other at pH 6.

Inulinase is activated when the pressed juice is treated with trypsin, pepsin, papain or pressed juice of the germinating shoot.

Jerusalem artichoke flowers mature late in fall and are a valuable source of nectar and pollen.

Sugar yield ranges from 0.09 to 0.3 mg/flower and honey production from 30-60 kg/hectare, in studies by Cirnu from Romania in 1988.

Recently, genetic engineers in Holland have altered the sugar beet by introducing genes from the Jerusalem artichoke. If this is commercially viable, it will change the economics of inulin as both beets and chicory use similar machinery and technology.

This creates a high tech sugar beet that produces fructan, instead of sucrose.

Fructans are polymers of fructose that cannot be digested by humans, and are therefore sought by low calorie food manufacturers.

Jerusalem artichoke naturally converts sucrose to fructan, and the genetically altered sugar beets grew normally and converted virtually all sucrose to fructans.

High fructose syrups are another possibility, with a greater sweetening effect than sucrose or D- glucose.

A fermented beer can be produced form the root sugars, and is said to be better than that from sugar beets.

Spring harvested tubers containing low molecular weight inulin are suited for fermentations or isolation of oligosaccharides; while fall harvested tubers not exposed to frost contain high molecular weight inulin and are better for production of high fructose syrup.

In China, the tubers are dried and pickled as a relish.

Both the tubers and tops can also be used for producing ethanol that is competitive with corn. During World War II, the French set up ten factories where fuel alcohol was made from Jerusalem Artichokes. One ton of tubers yielded 19 gallons of alcohol. The residue was then used as cattle feed. Bio ethanol is another possible application.

Several cultivars have been examined at Morden Research Station in Manitoba for production, including Columbia, Challenger and Sunroot 1000, which has red-colored roots.

Average yields of 16,000-20,000 kilos per hectare can be expected, with production costs similar to potatoes. At a conversion rate of 80-90%, ethanol yields of 3900-4500 litres per hectare could be achieved. This translates into 1.7, 2.0 and 3.7 times more alcohol per hectare than sugar beets, corn and wheat respectively.

While processing for ethanol, the protein can be extracted. Work by Curt et al, *Ind Crops and Products* 2006 24:3 found the potential of stems for bio-ethanol was 38% that of the tubers.

Content of sucrose and FOS has been found highest in the stalk in August, at least when grown in Norway. Slimestad et al, *J Sci Food* Ag 90:6.

And as a bonus, it has been found that roots grown in nematode infested soil can reduce the population by 45%, in studies by Kay in 1973.

Jerusalem Artichoke juice has been found to provide the same protection for weaner pigs as in feed as antibiotics. For two weeks after weaning, four ml of juice daily were recommended, and two hours after the meals, the lactic acid concentrations in the hindgut showed no increase.

Flower infusions have been used to kill flies. Tests have also shown that water infusions of the flowers are toxic to mice but not to rabbits.

An old remedy for baldness involved rubbing a cut tuber on the hair roots.

Fuseau, or tophinol, is thought to be a cross species hybrid of Jerusalem Artichoke and the Wood Sunflower (*H. strumosus*). This has not been substantiated, however. Fuseau, shaped like a spindle, is a popular cultivar, due to its easy peeling shape.

Breeding specialists have used hybridization to breed resistance into its close cousin, the sunflower. In fact, the two will produce fertile offspring.

MEDICINAL

CONSTITUENTS- sunflower seeds- high in Vit A B D (92 IU/100 g) and E, zinc, protein (24%), oil (47%), albumin, betaine, calcium, chlorine, flourine (2.6 ppm), copper, choline, histidine, iron, lecithin, as well as fatty acids; quinic and isochlorogenic, citric, tartaric, caffeic, and chlorogenic acids; SAM (S-adenosyl-methionine), Urease; helianthic acid; 270 mg/100 grams of phytosterols, composed mainly of beta sitosterol and lesser amounts of campesterol and stigmasterol. Trehalose is a unique sugar.

Seed sprouts- vitamin D

flowers- bisdesmosidic triterpenoid saponins (helianthosides), lutein (dried petal, 0.078%), sterols, syn alkane-6,8-diol; maniladiol, 24-methyl-enecyclo-artenol

sepal- sterol like substance (C21H3602)

corolla- 0.266% quercimeritrin.

root- inulin

young plants- asparagin, potassium nitrate, potassium carbonate, tannins, quercimetrin (flavonic glycoside).

leaf- citric and malic acid (1mg/gram), as well as malonic, lactic, succinic, aconitic, chlorogenic and fumaric acids, urease; heliannuols, three 7,10-heliannanes, nevadensin, a natural aglycone lignan, tanegool, as well as pinoresinol, lariciresinol, and di-hydro-dehydroiconiferilic alcohol.

pith- uronic acid (galacturonic complex). quinic and chlorogenic acids; as well as 53% sugars; potassium nitrate, potassium carbonate

receptacle- benzopyran derivatives.

galls- histopine

pollen- 8 fatty acid esters of triterpene alcohols, 4 free triterpene alcohols, 4 diterpene acids, six 3,4-seco-tirucallane-type triterpenoids, two tocopherol compounds, 4 estolides, 3 syn-alkane-4,6 diols; 1,3-dioxalkanoic acid, and an aliphatic ketone, and free fatty acids.

H. tuberosa- polysaccharides, in particular inulin (fructosan), diterpene acids, saccharose, pseudo-inulin, inulenin, helianthenin, synanthrin and a volatile oil including some beta bisabolen. The ripe tubers also contain levulose and dextrose, and 0.008% betaine hydrochloride.

Glutamine is the richest amino acid at 27.8 g/100 grams of protein. Also contains iron, silicon, and spermine.

stem- 14% cellulose.

leaves- deactylviquiestenin, erioflorin, chlorogenic acid

H. couplandii- kauranoic acid esters

H. nuttallii leaf- grandifloric acid, ciliaric acid, furanoheliangolides; 12,8-cis-lactonized eudesmanolides

H. petiolaris- leaves and flower heads- 5 kaurane and trachylobane type diterpenes, four 3,10-furanoheliango-lides; 5,10-epoxygermacranolide helivy-polide; 11alpah, 13-dihydrooxyde-hidrocostus lactone; the unusual 5,10-epoxy-germacranolide; and 3-methoxy-1,2-anhydridoniveusin A; niveusin B; ciliaric acid.

H. maximilianii- cumambranolide-8- (angelate); (2',3'-epoxyangelate); (2'-hydroxyethyl)acrylate; and sarracinate; 3-hydroxycostunolide-8-sarracinate; 2-hydroxycostunolide-8-(2',3'-epoxyange-late); desacetyl-eupasserin; tifruiticin; acetyl-tifruiticin; mollisorin B; deoxy-tifruiticin; acetyledeoxy-tifruiticin; an orizabin derivative; and an ent-labdane diterpene acid.

Sunflower seed and leaf infusions are used as a mild expectorant, useful for bronchial and laryngeal complaints. At one time roasted seed infusions were used for whooping cough. For asthma, the boiled seeds are decocted to half water and made into honey syrup.

The seeds combine well with comfrey and licorice root for this purpose.

A 1:10 tincture of the flower, made with 70% alcohol, is a recommended febrifuge.

Sunflower seeds are good for the muscles, nerves and blood vessels. The seeds are rich in arginine, an amino acid deficient in men with low sperm count. Arginine has potential cardiovascular health benefits, and is a precursor to nitric oxide.

Habitual eating of the seeds is said to build up physical endurance and resistance against disease. They are deficient in lysine, and when the seeds or flour is supplemented with lysine is a more complete protein, practically equal to that of casein. Sunflower seed combined with grain is a complete protein, high in biological food value.

They are said to help preserve natural sight for a long time without glasses.

Sunflower seeds contain SAM-e (S-adenosyl methionine) a compound used today for treating depression.

SAM-e has pain relieving and anti-inflammatory properties similar to ibuprofen. Much weaker, of course, it would take 250 grams of seed to equal the effect of a single dose of ibuprofen. One study of 20,641 patients with osteoarthritis found SAM-e as effective as OTC pain relievers. Berger & Nowak, *Am J Med* 1987 83.

Furthermore there are very few side effects. A two-year study by Konig, in the same journal, found no significant side effects.

It appears that SAMe increases chondrocyte activity, which involves destroying old cartilage to make room for new, or recycling and renewing. It also increases concentrations of synovial fluid 3-4 times, helping lubricate joints.

It prevents the breakdown of proteoglycans, cartilage molecules that retain water, and make the joints flexible and moist.

Najm and other researchers at U of California, Irvine *BMC Musculoskel Disord* 2004 5:1 found "SAMe…is as effective as celecoxib in the management of the symptoms of knee osteoarthritis". In this randomized, double-blind crossover study, researchers assigned 56 patients either 1200 mg of SAMe or 200 mg celecoxib daily for four months. The drug works more quickly, but SAMe was found equally effective over time.

SAMe undergoes methylation and during breakdown releases homocysteine, which can cause cardiovascular harm. In the presence of B vitamins, especially B6, B12, and folic acid, the homocysteine re-methylates into methionine or is converted to glutathione, a useful anti-oxidant. Fortunately, sunflower seeds are rich in B vitamins.

Sunflower seeds are a rich source of phenylalanine, which helps reduce pain by inhibiting the breakdown of enkephalins, chemicals involved in pain perception. In laboratory rats, phenylalanine enhanced the effect of morphine and prolonged its action. In humans, it makes acupuncture for reducing pain more effective.

It is involved in the methylation of monoamines, neurotransmitters and phospholipids.

Normally, the brain manufactures all the SAMe it needs from methionine, but in depressed patients the synthesis is impaired. Added SAMe results in increased production of serotonin and dopamine, and improved binding of neuro-transmitters to receptor sites.

Matthew Wood notes that sunflowers are Bear medicine. The root is brown and furry, and the seeds contain oils that build up the adrenals and kidneys.

Sunflower kernels contain choline, lecithin and betaine, the latter reducing homocysteine levels in the blood and protecting against heart disease. Choline and lecithin are precursors to phospholipids needed to nourish and insulate neurons of the body and brain.

Betaine is a minor component of red wine, and yet may be part of the French Paradox of a highly saturated fat diet, and low national cardiovascular disease rates. Betaine is rich in beets (see Liver) and is a pre-cursor of dopamine production.

Sunflower seed proteins, when hydrolyzed with pepsin and pancreatin, are a potential source of ACE inhibitory peptide. Inhibition of the angiotensin-I converting enzyme leads to reduction of hypertension. Cristina Megias et al, *J Ag Food Chem* 2004 52 suggested defatted sunflower meal may be a useful supplement source of bioactive peptides with anti-hypertensive properties.

Secoisolariciresinol, a lignan also found in flaxseed, with activity both phytoestrogenic and anti-oxidant, is found in sunflower seeds, but in much lower amounts.

Sunflower seeds in a water extract have been found to exhibit anti-asthmatic benefit, *in vivo*. Work by Heo et al, *Int J Mol Med* 2008 21:1 found the extract decreased CD4+ and IgE levels, and changed the IL-4/IL-13 expression in mice.

The seeds are rich in chlorogenic and caffeic acids, anti-oxidants with anti-carcinogenic activity.

A derivative of chlorogenic acid from sunflower seed is an inhibitor of arginase and the seeds also contain trypsin enzyme inhibitors.

Work by Moller et al, *Phytother Res* 2008 Nov 11 found ethanol extracts of sunflower and flax seeds possess strong lipase inhibition.

The pectin found in seeds helps give protection against radiation poisoning, according to Dr. Eugene Zampieron and Ellen Kamhi, in *The Natural Medicine Chest*. Not sure.

The seeds contain a unique sugar, trehalose, previously known as mushroom sugar or mycose. It is found naturally in sugars produced by Douglas fir and other conifers.

In Huntington's disease, a huntingtin protein binds to a transcription regulator within a cell, and the genetic activity is disturbed and the cell's control of protein synthesis breaks down. This leads to glutamate remaining between neurons, acting as an excitotoxin.

The elongated huntingtin protein chain causes the neurons to kill themselves.

In 2004, researchers at the RIKEN Brain Science Institute inhibited the aggregation of the proteins with trehalose. This blocking of clumping delayed the disease's onset in mice. Harper et al, *Proceed Nat Acad Sci* 2005 102 16.

Sunflower seed sprouts are a rich source of vitamin D, and high in antioxidant activity.

The sprouts contain high levels of cynarin, and exhibit inhibition of advanced glycation end products, in a manner stronger than aminoquandine. Sun, Z et al, *J Ag Food Chem* 2012 60:12 3260-5.

In Traditional Chinese Medicine, the sunflower seed is decocted to treat constipation, and to promote eruption of measles. It is known as either **XIANG RI KUI ZI** meaning facing sun flower seed; **YI ZHANG JU**, meaning ten foot chrysanthemum, or simply **KUI HUA ZI**.

Dr. Cook considered sunflower seed, burdock seed and Bittersweet (*Celastrus scandens*) to be the only remedies that effectively increase sebaceous sweat from the skin.

The sunflower seed shells are used for tinnitus in the form of a decoction.

The leaves are considered bitter, stomachic and useful for treating high blood pressure.

The stems can be cut and dried and infused for intermittent fevers, and are diuretic and useful in inflammatory conditions of the urinary tract.

The flower receptacle is used in folk medicine in China and known as **HSIANG JIH KUEI HUA PAN**.

It is decocted for its sweet, warm property and used to promote urination, reduce heat of headaches, dizziness and toothache.

The flowers are used for stomach and abdominal pain, inducing labour and menorrhagia.

Ethanol extracts of the flower head have been shown to reduce blood pressure in cats, due to the dilation of blood vessels.

The flower petals contain syn-alkane-6, 8-diol, shown to inhibit tumour promoting activity and possess remarkable anti-inflammatory activity. Ukiya et al, *J Agric Food Chemistry* 2003 51.

Flower petals of *H. angustifolia* exhibit activity against leukemia, breast, glioblastoma, and colon cancer cell lines. Kretschmer et al, *Planta Med* 77:17 1912-15

Sunflower pollen showed potent inhibitory effect, 97-100%, on Epstein-Barr virus early antigen, in the same study. In a later study in *J Nat Products* 66:11 the author identified sunpollenol and other 3,4-seco tricallan type triterpenoids in the flowers.

The fresh roots are used for treating stomachache, urinary problems, constipation, traumatic injury, and hernias. In southern China, the fresh root is decocted for treating pain in the penis due to gonorrhea. For hernias, the decoction is mixed with brown sugar.

The pith is used for urinary troubles, including milky or bloody urine, as well as stones. It is used for treating whooping cough and external bleeding.

For stones of the urethra or kidney, a meter of pith is slowly boiled down to one quarter of original volume and taken once daily for one week.

In Mongolia, the fresh pith is mashed and applied directly to wounds and cuts to stop bleeding.

The flower receptacles are decocted to treat headaches, dizziness, toothache, stomachache, menstrual pain, sores and swellings.

Recently in China, the fresh receptacles have been boiled until a sticky mass remains. This is applied to affected arthritic joints with all patients showing some improvement.

For mastitis, the receptacles are cleaned of seeds, and dried, chopped and roasted until powder. Nine to 16 grams are mixed in white wine, with all 122 patients reporting satisfactory results.

Helianthoside A, a bitter saponin from the petals, has been shown hemolytic.

In Russia, the seeds are used for bronchial infections, and the stems and heads macerated in vodka (what else?) for tuberculosis and malaria.

In Italy, the aerial parts are used as a diuretic, febrifuge and stimulant.

The well-strained water can be used to ease acute eye inflammation.

The whole plant can be decocted and added to bath water for arthritic pain and joint swelling.

The crushed root is applied to bruises. Heated, the roots relieve rheumatism; when applied cold are good for blisters and headaches.

The root contains inulin, which scientific research has shown to be effective against the wheezing associated with asthma and other bronchial conditions.

Early Eclectic physicians, such as Dr. Howard suggested western sunflower root for medicinal purpose. "A strong decoction of the root, drank freely, will operate as an emetic, and by continuing its used more moderately, relaxes the bowels, promotes perspiration, and effectually cures fevers."

Medicinally, the seed oil is specific for coughs as well as inflammation of the bladder and diseases of the kidney.

Sunflower leaves are astringent in nature, and have been infused for intermittent fever associated with malaria and other such conditions, and confirmed by Danzel.

This may be explained, in part, by the fact that flower infusions have weak insecticidal properties.

The green leaves and stems show positive for *Staphylococcus aureus*, while the roots show activity against *Micrococcus tuberculosis.*

Trachlboban-19-oic acid and (-)-kaur-16-en-19-oic acid are both anti-microbial agents in the Sunflower.

Laboratory tests indicate that flower extracts are very stimulating to intestinal contraction, and may be of use in intestinal atony.

Nevadensin is found in the leaves and glandular trichomes of several Sunflower species. The compound shows activity against tuberculosis at the rate of 0.2 mg/ml-1 *in vitro*. Reddy GB et al, *Int J Pharmacognosy* 1991 29.

The same study found significant anti-inflammatory and cytotoxic activity. The compound was more effective than wogonin (see Scullcap) in Dalton's lymphoma and Ehrlich ascites carcinoma cells. Dong et al, *J Nat Prod* 1987 50.

Nevadensin exhibits hypotensive effects, both central and peripheral, in nature. Song et al, *Acta Pharm Sin* 1985 6.

It exhibits activity against *Escherichia coli* and *Staphylococcus aureus*. Brahmachari et al, *Open Nat Prod Journal* 2008 1. A more complete review of nevadensin can be found by same author in *Int J Green Pharm* 2010 4:4.

Niveusin C, in common and narrow-leaved Sunflower, has proven cytotoxic and anti-tumour activity.

Sunflower, like nettles and spinach, contains choline acetyltransferase, a form of acetylcholine for the brain.

Triterpenoid saponins derived from sunflower, Plohmann et al, U of Regensburg, Germany (1997), showed immune-modulating and anti-tumour effect.

Helianol, a triterpene alcohol present in *H. annuus* flowers showed marked anti-inflammatory activity. Akihisa et al, Nihon University in Tokyo, 1996.

Cosmos, safflower and Chinese chrysanthemum all contain, interestingly enough, some helianol.

Sunflower petals contain maniladiol and other compounds that reduce inflammatory response. Other triterpene glycosides may also be responsible for anti-inflammatory properties. Ukiya et al, *J Nat Prod* 70:5.

The sunflower receptacles have been analyzed for anti-microbial substances. Satoh et al, Hokkaido University, Japan, 1996. Two anti-fungal benzopyran derivatives have been isolated and evaluated.

In the mesophyll cells of sunflower cotyledons, are found high catalase concentrations.

Crown gall tumours on sunflower contain histopine, an unusual amino acid derivative of histidine.

Jerusalem Artichokes are a medicinal food, rich in inulin, a sugar without need for insulin, and suitable for diabetes, atherosclerosis, and obesity diets.

Jerusalem Artichokes can be juiced, for example, along with carrot, beets, celery and other vegetables that satisfy "our sweet tooth", and satiate flavor centers of the brain, by triggering taste buds on the sides of the tongue. This is very helpful in weight loss programs, where the brain is constantly seeking pleasurable foods.

Work by Burkova et al, in 2004 studied the tuber powder in a controlled study on obese spa patients. Studies found those patients taking the powder improved their carbohydrate and lipid metabolism as well as blood and hormonal factors such as cortisol, thyroxin, and insulin.

Fructooligosaccharides (FOS) present in the tubers has been found to enhance and promote the growth of healthy bacteria in the human intestine. This is significant and could be a very helpful tool, in those immune compromised individuals needing to restore normal bowel flora.

Inulin derivatives possess anti-arrhythmic, anti-tuberculosis, anti-carcinogenic, anti-coagulating, and fibrinolytic properties.

Dr. Vogel suggests that the tincture is "favorable to men's libido and to the production of spermatozoids".

The leaf and stalk can be prepared as an infusion for the relief of rheumatism. Afro-Americans of South Carolina steeped the leaves in rum as a remedy for dropsy, and kidney tonic.

Both the stem and root give positive antibacterial results against various gram positive and negative bacteria like *Staphylococcus aureus* and *E. coli*.

The leaves contain chlorogenic acid, which has a structure similar to the anti-viral, anti-flu drugs Tamiflu and Relenza.

The plant is known as Topinambour, in France and parts of Europe. In 1613, six natives from the Topinambous tribe of Brazil were brought to the court of King Louis XIII. The new vegetable had just been introduced but lacking a novel name, put the two together, figuring they both came from the same part of the New World.

A recent paper by Bobrovnyk et al, from Kiev, was delivered at a *Precision Agricultural and Biological Control* conference in Boston in 1998. It articulates other medicinal and bioactive substances in the plant. Spermine, for example, is used in biochemical research.

Experiments by Reshetnik et al, *Voprosy-Pitaniya* 1998 1 found that the tubers have very low ability to absorb heavy metals, including lead, cobalt, nickel, strontium, and caesium.

A list of possible applications of inulin from Jerusalem artichoke include prebiotics, dietary fibre, sweeteners, high fructose syrups, and purified inulin for medical use.

Non-food uses include furfural, mannitol, glycerol, ethylene glycol, acetone, butanol, succinic acid, lactic acid and a range of complexing agents for precipitation of heavy metals.

Ten patents for medical/veterinary application have been filed, including treatment of calcium deficiency, diabetic hepatosis, synanthrin (blood stabilizer), as well as a cell growth factor with anti-tumor and anti-cancer activity.

As of 2008, over 150 applications for use in food, drink and nutraceuticals have been filed, as well as animal feeds and various industrial uses.

The book by Kays and Nottingham in the bibliography is a definitive text on this plant.

HOMEOPATHY

Sunflower (*H. annuus*) is used in cases of intermittent fever. It is for nasal congestion, catarrh, as well as nasal hemorrhage and thick scabs of the nose.

It is specific to rheumatic pain of the left knee, and is used externally as a vulnerary like Arnica and Calendula.

It is indicated for vomiting, black stools, congestion of the mouth and pharynx, and redness and heat of the skin.

The symptoms are aggravated by heat and relieved by vomiting. It is considered a spleen remedy, with marked effect on the stomach, whenever there is nausea and vomiting, and dry mouth.

DOSE- Tincture and low potencies. The mother tincture is prepared from the freshly and coarsely powdered seeds.

These provings are based on two males and one female taking expressed juice of the flowers and one woman eating excessive amounts of seeds in 1848.

Jerusalem Artichoke (*H. tuberosa*) is used for constipation, obesity, and as a therapeutic aid in the treatment of diabetes mellitus.

It is also helpful in helping achieve gradual weight loss without the rebound effect. It curbs the appetite and provides a source of energy at the same time.

DOSE- Mother tincture and low potency. Intake of larger quantities of the partially hydrolyzed pressed must (with its high fructose content) can lead to elevated serum triglyceride levels in men.

Quantities that exceed 50 grams of fructose per day should be avoided, particularly in cases of hyper-triglyceridaemia or kidney insufficiency.

SEED OIL

Traditional sunflower seed oil is 69% linoleic acid. Hybrid breeding is changing all that, however.

Oleic acid is a monosaturated fatty acid that can lower serum cholesterol and the risk of coronary heart disease.

NuSun hybrids, mentioned above, can produce oil with nearly 30% less saturated fatty acids than traditional hybrids. Potato chips fried in such an oil could be labeled as low in saturated fat.

Mid-oleic oils (60-75%) require no hydrogenation and are low in saturated fats, creating new demand in the marketplace.

The costly and unhealthy step of bubbling hydrogen into polyunsaturated oils- partial hydrogenation won’t be required to protect against flavour deterioration.

No hydrogenation means no trans-fatty acids that are harmful to health.

The sunflower oil can be used internally to relieve constipation, acting as a lubricant. It can also be used externally as massage oil, or for poorly healing wounds in the form of an oil dressing. Numerous cosmetic companies, including Revlon, L'Oreal, Clairol, Avon and Vaseline, use sunflower seed oil in gels, creams, and hair product formulas.

It has been used in the past for skin sores, rheumatism and psoriasis.

Sunflower oil is an effective diuretic and can help to build healthy teeth in young children. Again, however, the quality of processing is all important. When oils were heated over 110° C, and fed to lab rats, the oil was found to cause liver damage and enhance effects of carcinogens.

A study was conducted by Prottey et al in 1975 on three patients suffering essential fatty acids due to chronic mal-absorption, and scaly dermatitis.

Cutaneous applications of sunflower seed oil to their right arms for two weeks led to major increases in the level of linoleic acids in the epidermal lecithin, significant lowering in the rate of transdermal water loss and the disappearance of scaly lesions.

Ozonized sunflower oil demonstrates significant anti-microbial activity as well as anti-inflammatory and wound healing problems. Topical application to preterm infants, in a randomized, controlled clinical trial, showed a significant reduction of nosocomical infections. Darnstadt et al, *Ped Infect Dis J* 2004 23.

Rodenas et al, *J Am Coll Nutr* 2005 24:5 found a mixture of sunflower and olive oil decreased total cholesterol, LDL and a lipoprotein in fourteen post menopausal women over four weeks. This suggests that a human trial of canola and sunflower oil may produce similar findings and a potential market opportunity.

Sunflower seed oil is a good substrate for production of CLA, or conjugated linoleic acid.

CLA is found naturally in milk, butter, cheese and meat, due to bacterial fermentation in the rumen, and is used in supplements, dietetic foods, as well as skin care and cosmetic products. Areas of interest include weight loss, and potential anti-cancer activity.

In Ayurvedic medicine, sunflower seed oil is held under the tongue for twenty minutes and then spit out. Matthew Wood mentions it is an old Cherokee recipe for alcohol poisoning. The mouth is later rinsed out to remove the toxins.

He writes of a client poisoned by dental work. He had her hold sunflower oil under the tongue three times daily. After about ten minutes, the oils was burning, the same effect caused by the dental materials, and then she spit it out. She continued until the burning stopped, tapered off and recovered.

Sunflower oil is a reliable source of mixed tocopherols of vitamin E, making it the only vitamin E containing beta sitosterols, stigmasterols and campesterols.

An interesting, unusual study by P. Whitten, *Biology of Reproduction* 1993 49 had rat mothers fed sunflower seed oil, rich in coumestrol. Transferred through milk to newborn pups, the estrogenic effect of only ten days profoundly affected ovulation and sterility in females, and less mounting and fewer ejaculations in the juvenile males.

Sunflower oil is an attractant to leaf cutting ants, and may be useful in poisonous traps.

Prairie Sunflower (*H. couplandii*) seed contains 30% oil composed mainly (65%) of linolenic acid, 26% oleic acid and 5% saturated fats.

Narrow-leaved Sunflower (*H. maximilianii*) seed contains 30% oil, with 73% linoleic, 13% oleic, and just 0.5% linolenic acid.

Wild sunflower seed oil, native to Canada, contain 6% saturated fats; half of Mexican.

LEAF, STEM & ROOT OIL

Jerusalem Artichoke contains lipids in all plant parts, consisting of fatty acids and unsaponifiable substances.

The leaves contain 2.7% lipids composed of 42% palmitic, 31% linoleic, 20% linolenic, and small amounts of oleic and stearic acids.

The stems contain 1.2% composed mainly of 45% palmitic and 40% linolenic acids.

The tubers contain 54% linoleic and 30% palmitic acid, as well as 12% linolenic.

The stem and leaf oil is dark green, that from the tubers a light brown.

ESSENTIAL OIL

The tubers of Jerusalem artichoke are said to contain volatile oil with beta-bisabolen. This should be investigated more thoroughly.

The sunflower heads contain 0.2% of a strong smelling essential oil, composed of 72.6% alpha pinene.

Gerard, in his famous English Herbal, wrote the sunflower centre is "like some curious cloth wrought with the needle… from which sweats forth excellent fine and clear turpentine". Parkinson added that in warm weather both the flowers and leaf joints "sweat out a fine thin and clear rosin or turpentine, so like clear Venice turpentine that it cannot be known from it".

And oleo-distillate of the seeds in a 2% ointment has been found useful in a trial involving 20 adults with atopic dermatitis. Eichanfield et al, *Pediatr Dermatol* 2009 26:6.

Sunflower leaf essential oil contains 23% sabinene, 28% alpha pinene, 12% limonene and 7.8% isobornylacetate.

WAX

A wax has been isolated from sunflower seed oil, and found to consist mainly of ceryl cerotate. The hulls contain up to 10% of the same wax.

Ceryl Cerotate melts at 84 C, with the formula C22H104O2. A minor part of the wax is sitosterol. It could be recovered from the whole sunflower seed with a solvent, before pressing, or later from the press cake.

Sunflower seed wax, if derived from supercritical fluid extraction, or another natural process, has use in the cosmetic industry.

Ching T. Hou, a chemist working in Peoria, Illinois found a *Pseudomonas aeruginosa*, growing in pond water, has the ability to convert the oleic acids in corn, safflower and sunflower oils into an unusual structure.

The compound called 7, 10-dihydroxy-8-(E)-octadecenoic acid is an excellent starting material for creating plastics, lubricants, paints, and new antibiotics.

FLOWER ESSENCES

Sunflower essence heals disturbances or distortions in the soul's relationship to the masculine. This is often associated with a conflicted or deficient relationship with the father in childhood. Sunflower essence brings to the soul the quality of light.

FLOWER ESSENCE SOCIETY

Sunflower essence is for compassion and tenderness; for the expressed love for helpless people, animals and the environment. It may be used with children who are selfish, or those who steep themselves in righteousness and superiority. Humility and inter-dependence are better understood. **NEW ZEALAND**

Jerusalem Artichoke essence helps in the recognition that the knowledge and experience of other people can be very valuable.

MIRIANA

Sunflower essence tempers and spiritualizes the male ego. Lessening the impact of the overbearing male ego awakens the male's maternal instinct and desire to have children. This draws the individual closer to a sense of androgyny within the self. It also aligns the superconscious mind's spiritual values with the heart chakra.

Sunflower balances the yin and yang energies, and attunes people to higher wisdom. People demonstrating anger or hostility towards their father experience increased understanding with this essence.

Osteopathic and chiropractic adjustments are augmented. It stimulates the kundalini and aligns it properly along the spine. On the cellular level, absorption of vitamin D increases.

Sunflower dissolves fatty tissue. The ability of plants to receive the afternoon or evening sun will be enhanced. **GURUDAS**

POLLEN ESSENCE

Sunflower pollen essence is for uplifting and strengthening. **HORUS**

SPIRITUAL PROPERTIES

Sunflower tempers and spiritualizes the male ego, and draws the individual closer to a sense of androgeny. It balances yin and yang energies, and attunes people to higher wisdom.

When people have trouble with their intuition, and want to know if their perception is correct, or if it is just the idle chatter of the material mind, sunflower resolves the problem.

On a cellular level, the absorption of Vitamin D is increased. It eases sunburn particularly if there is heat exhaustion or toxicity in the skin, including skin cancer.

Sunflower dissolves fatty tissue.

Associations with Leo are noted, for instance, the ability of individuals to work with progressed energy through Leo. **GURUDAS**

These petals are an uncompromising yellow-orange. The color seems to contain all the energy this planet will ever need. This color could power a nuclear reactor. It rings like a carillon. It hits me, with a little punch, in the solar plexus. **RUSSELL**

PERSONALITY TRAITS

The Sunflower originated in the New World, so any mention of sunflower in ancient Greece probably pertains to a daisy or marigold type flower that turns and follows the sun across the sky.

The Greeks called the Sunflower, Clytie or Kleite (Famous One).

Classical writers made her a water nymph who loved the sun god and followed his fructifying beams with her head. Since her name was also the root of the word Clitoris (Kleitoris), it seems that the myth may have begun with symbols of the divine marriage between Father Heaven and Mother Earth. **WALKER**

Helios was born of Euryphaessa, the Moon Goddess, and the Titan Hyperion, who fathered Selene and the dawn goddess Eos.

In mythology, Helios was drowned by the Titans at sea, but rose up and ascended into the sky. Helios had a magnificent eastern palace that he left every morning and arrived in the western Islands of the Blessed every evening. He and his horses rested that night, and a golden ferry fashioned by Hephaestus, the Smith God, carried him, via the river Oceanus back east to start the journey anew.

In myth, he had a single round eye with which he observed everything.

PRAIRIE DEVA

When I hear Jerusalem, I think of a spiritual place, the Bible's holy land; a place close to God that exudes purity and intimacy. In good Christian conscience I would like to change the name of this vegetable to Siberian Artichoke, or Dark side of the Moon Artichoke.

DARYL SHEPPARD

DOCTRINE OF SIGNATURES

The deep root system of sunflower is far reaching, giving it the ability to draw trace minerals that may not be found in the topsoil.

The flower head's ability to follow the sun throughout the day is also a signature of the plant's amazing talents. Along with the vitamins and other nutrients found in sunflower seeds, these signatures symbolize the wealth of nutrients the plant has to offer us, and its incredible relationship with the sun.

The golden-yellow colour and shape of flower head, along with the golden yellowish, purplish disk, is also symbolic of the sun, and represent the fire of life, the will.

The stalk is sturdy and tall and gives a feeling of great strength, endurance, and a desire to reach toward the sun's natural power and light. These signatures relate to the third chakra, will, purpose, power, self-empowerment, and self honour. This is the energy centre that gives us the ability to think and reason, to gather the strength and power from deep within our roots, to find purpose and desire in life, to empower ourselves with who we are.The third chakra or solar plexus centre is sun energy. It is associated with the left side of the brain and its activities, representing the male or yang energy.

This gives us the ability to assert ourselves in the world with positive determination, optimism, and direction.The sunflower's large disk represents an eye. The eye of this plant is open wide and offers a journey of seeing and believing. **PALLASDOWNEY**

MYTHS AND LEGENDS

The people of India used the flower to represent their sun god Surya, and the people of ancient Persia used it to represent their sun god Mithras.

RECIPES

SUNBUTTER- Take one cup of raw sunflower seeds and add 1 2 tbsp of honey, or rosehips syrup and blend. Refrigerate. The seeds contain over 50% protein and are suitable for those needing to put on weight. It is a very rich spread not suitable for weight watchers!

SUNFLOWER SEED CHEESE- In the evening, take one pound of raw, shelled sunflower seeds, and cover with distilled water. In the morning, drain and combine one cup of soaked seeds, with one cup of distilled water, and put into blender or food processor. Pour into large bowl and let set for 4-7 hours. When ready, the surface will be puffy, and the water will have separated from puree, with a mild yogurt like smell.

Strain through cheesecloth, and then tie up corners and squeeze to remove excess moisture. Stored in fridge, it will keep about one week.

Use as a vegetable dip, or sandwich spread. As the protein, fats, and sugars are all predigested, the cheese is a very balanced and nutritious food.

CHOKE COFFEE- Slice the washed, fresh roots and place on cookie sheet. Slow roast in oven at 250° F, until dark brown. Grind and use as coffee substitute.

SUNFLOWER BATH Take whole dried plant, including some stem, and decoct until a beautiful purple gold. This is strained and added to hot baths for rheumatic and arthritic pain.

ABOUT THE AUTHOR

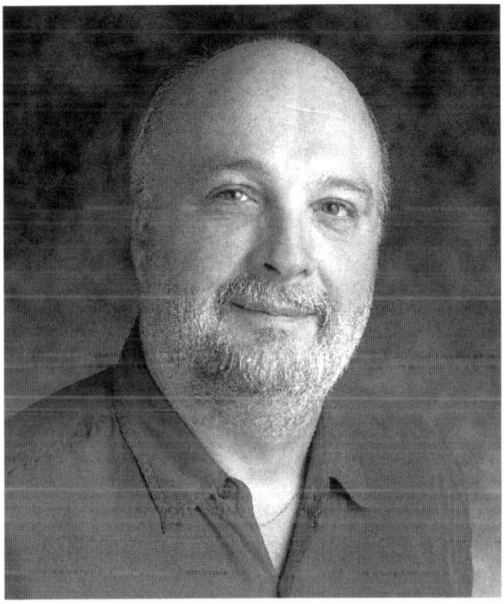

Robert Dale Rogers has been an herbalist for over forty years. He has a Bachelor of Science from the University of Alberta, where he is an assistant clinical professor in Family Medicine. He teaches plant medicine, including herbology and flower essences at Grant MacEwan University, as well as Earth Spirit Medicine at the Northern Star College of Mystical Studies in Edmonton, Alberta, Canada.

Robert is past chair of the Alberta Natural Health Agricultural Network and Community Health Council of Capital Health. He is a Fellow of the International College of Nutrition, chair of the medicinal mushroom committee of the North American Mycological Association and on the editorial board of the International Journal of Medicinal Mushrooms, and Discovery Phytomedicine.

Robert co-hosts The Alberta Herb Gathering held every second year (www.albertaherbgathering.com)

He lives on Millcreek Ravine in Edmonton with his beautiful and talented wife, Laurie Szott-Rogers and out of control cat Ceres.

You can email him at scents@telusplanet.net
or visit
www.selfhealdistributing.com

BIBLIOGRAPHY

Abbe, Elfriede, The Fern Herbal, Cornell University Press, Ithaca, 1981
Acorn, J. Bugs of Alberta, Lone Pine Publishing, Edmonton, AB, 2000.
Adams, J. Les Plantes Medicinales. Bulletin 23, Agriculture Canada. 1916
Adams, Jean. Insect Potpourri, Adventures in Entomology. Sandhill Crane Press, FL. 1992
Aggarwal, Bharat. Healing Spices. Sterling Pub. New York 2011.
Albert-Puleo, Michael. Economic Botany, 32, Jan-Mar, 1978.
Allaby, Michael. Temperate Forests. Facts on File. New York. 1999.
Allen, D & Hatfield, G. Medicinal Plants in Folk Tradition. Timber Press, Portland. 2004
Allen,E, Morrison,D, &Wallis,G. Common Tree Diseases of B.C. Canada Forest Service, '96
Allende, Isabel. Aphrodite- A Memoir of the Senses. Harper Flamingo. New York. 1998.
Alstat, Ed. Electic Dispensatory of Botanical Therapeutics. Ecl Med. Oregon. 1989.
Anderson, Anne, Some Native Herbal Remedies, Pub 8A, Devonian Botanical Gardens 1980
_____ Plants in Cree. Duval House Pub. Edmonton AB 2000.
Anderson, C.&Tischer,T. Poinsettias, the December Flower, Waters Edge Press, CA, 1997
Andoh, Anthony. The Science & Romance of Selected Herbs used in Medicine and Religious Ceremony. North Scale Institute. San Francisco. 1986.
Andre, Alestine & Fehr, Alan. Gwich'in Ethnobotany. Gwich'in Social and Cultural Institute, Box 46, Tsiigehtchie, NWT, X0E 0B0, fax 1867-953-3820.
Andrews, Tamra. Nectar and Ambrosia. ABC-CLIO Box 1911 Santa Barbara CA. 2000.
Andrews, Ted. Animal Speak- The Spiritual and Magical Powers, Llewellyn. Minn. 1996.
_____ Animal Wise, DragonHawk, Jackson, TN, 1999.
Antol, Marie. The Incredible Secrets of Mustard. Avery Pub. New York. 1999.
Aronson J K Ed. Meyler's Side Effects of Herbal Medicines. Elsevier Amsterdam. 2009.
Arrowsmith, Nancy. Essential Herbal Wisdom. Llewellyn Pub. Woodbury, Minn. 2009.
Arsdall, Anne Van. Medieval Herbal Remedies. Routledge, New York. 2002.
Arvigo & Balick, Rainforest Remedies, Lotus Press, Twin Lakes, WI. 1993
Arvigo & Epstein. Rainforest Home Remedies, Harper SanFrancisco, 2001.
Assiniwi, Bernard. La Medecine des Indiens d' Amerique, Guerin Literature, 1988
Atal C.K. & Kapur B. Cultivation and Utilization of Medicinal Plants, Jammu-Tawi, 1982
Attenborough, David. The Private Life of Plants. Princeton U Press. Princeton NJ 1995.
Ausubel, K. Seeds of Change The Living Treasure. HarperSanFrancisco, 1994.
Aversano, Laura. The Divine Nature of Plants. Swan•Raven & Co. Columbus, NC, 2002.
Ayensu, Edward,S. Medicinal Plants of the West Indies, Reference Publications, 1981
Baïracli Levy, Juliette Herbal Handbook for Farm and Stable, Faber&Faber, London, 1952
Baker, Phil. The Dedalus Book of Absinthe. Dedalus 2001.
Barl, Branka et al, Saskatchewan Herb Database, U. of Sask. Saskatoon, 1996.
Barlow, Max. From the Shepherd's Purse. 1990
Barnes J, Anderson L, &Phillipson J. Herbal Medicines, A guide for healthcare professionals. Pharmaceutical Press, London, 2002.
Barnett, Robert A. Tonics, Harper Collins, New York, N.Y. 1997
Bartram, Thomas. Bartram's Encyl. of Herbal Medicine, Robinson Pub. London, 1998.
Bascom, Angella. Incorporating Herbal Medicine into Clinical Practice. F. Davis Co. 2002
Beals, Katherine, M. Flower Lore and Legend, Henry Holt, 1917
Beers, Susan-Jane. Jamu The ancient Indonesian Art of Herbal Healing, Periplus, 2001.
Belcourt, Christi. Medicines to Help Us. Gabriel Dumont Instit. Saskatoon, SK 2007.
Béliveau, R & Gingras,D. Foods That Fight Cancer. McClelland & Stewart Toronto. 2006.
Belsinger S & Dille C. Cooking with Herbs. CBI- Van Nostrand Reinhold, N.Y. 1984.

Benjamin, D.R. Mushrooms: Poisons and Panaceas. WH Freeman, San Francisco, 1995.
Bennet, Doug & Tiner, Tim. Up North. Reed Books Canada. Markham, Ont. 1993.
_____ Up North Again. McClelland and Stewart. Toronto, 1997.
Bennet, J & Rowley S. Uqalurait An Oral History of Nunavut. McGill Queens, Mont. 2004
Benyus, Janine. Biomimicry Innovation Inspired by Nature. William Morrow. 1997.
Berenbaum,May R. Buzzwords, A Scientists Muses on Sex, Bugs and Rock N Roll, Joseph Henry Press, Washington, D.C. 2000.
_____ Bugs in the System. Helix Books, Addison-Wesley Pub. 1995.
Beresford-Kroeger, Diana. The Global Forest. Viking Penguin. 2010.
_____ Arboretum Borealis. U Michigan Press. 2010.
Berliocchi,Luigi. The Orchid in Lore and Legend. Timber Press, Portland Oregon, 2000.
Berlund B & Bolsby C. The Edible Wild Pagurian Press, Toronto, Ont. 1971.
Berkowsky, Bruce. Mount Julius Flower Remedies. Mt. Vernon Washington, 1986
Bermejo, J & Leon,J. Neglected Crops-1492 ... FAO Series 26, United Nations, Rome, 1994.
Bernhardt, P. The Rose's Kiss, A Natural History of Flowers . Island Press, Covelo CA 1999
Bianchi, Ivo. Geriatrics and Homotoxicology. Aurelia-Verlag GmbH, Baden Baden, 1994.
Bianchini, F. The Complete Book of Health Plants. Crescent Books, New York, 1975.
Biship, Carol. The Book of Home Remedies &Herbal Cures, Jonathan-James, Toronto, 1979.
Bisset, Norman G. Herbal Drugs and Phytopharmaceuticals. 2nd Ed. CRC Press, 2001.
Blackburn, Thomas. December's Child: A Book of Chumash Oral Narratives , U of California Press, Berkeley, 1975.
Blanchan, Neltje. Nature's Garden. Doubleday, Page&Co. New York, 1900.
Bland, John. Forests of Liliput. Prentice Hall, Englewood Cliffs, New Jersey, 1971.
Bliss, Anne. Rocky Mountain Dye Plants. Juniper House, Boulder, Colorado, 1976
Blouin, Glen. Weeds of the Woods. Goose Lane, Fredericton, New Brunswick 1992.
_____ An Eclectic Guide to Trees, east of the Rockies. Boston Mills, 2001.
Boas, F. Ethnology of the Kwakiutl. Bureau of Am. Ethnology, 35th annual report, 1921.
Boericke, Wm. Materia Medica with Repetory. B. Jain Publishers. 1976
Boik, John. Natural Compunds in Cancer Therapy. Oregon Med Press, Princeton,Minn 2001
Boland, Bridget. Gardener's Magic &Other Old Wives' Lore. The Bodley Head, London, 77.
Bolton, Brett L. The Secret Powers of Plants. Berkley Pub Co. New York. 1974.
Bolton, J.L. Alfalfa, Botany, Cultivation &Utilization. Interscience Pub, New York, 1962.
Bone, Kerry. A Clinical Guide to Blending Liquid Herbs. Churchill Livingstone. 2003
Borrel, Marie. Healing Plants. Cassell & Co. Wellington House, London. 2001.
Bouchardon, Patrice. The Healing Energies of Trees. Journey Editions, Boston, 1999.
Bossenmaier, Eugene. Mushrooms of the Boreal Forest. U. of Saskatchewan Press, 1997
Boulos, Loutfy. Medicinal Plants of North Africa, Reference Pub. Algonac, Mich. 1983
Bowles, E. Joy. The Chemistry of Aromatherapeutic Oils. Allen & Unwin, Crow's Nest, Australia, 2003.
Bowman, Daria. Hydrangeas. Friedman/Fairfax Pub. New York. 1999.
Bradley, Peter. British Herbal Compendium Vol 2 Brit Herb Med Assoc. Bournemouth 2006.
Brahmachari, Goutam Ed. Natural Products, Alpha Sci Int Ltd. Oxford UK 2009.
Brandeis, Gayle. Fruitflesh. Harper Collins, San Francisco. 2002.
Brennan, M. Complete Holistic Care & Healing for Horses. Trafalgar Sq. Pub. VT. 2001.
Bringhurst, Robert. A Story as Sharp as a Knife. Douglas&McIntyre Vancouver, 1999.
Brinker, Francis N.D. Herb Contraindications and Drug Interactions .Third Edition Eclectic Medical Publications, Sandy, Oregon, 2001
_____ The Toxicology of Botanical Medicines, revised 2nd. Eclectic Med, Oregon, 1996.
_____ Eclectic Dispensatory of Botanical Therapeutics, Vol 2, Ecl. Med . Oregon, 1995.
Brodo, Irwin & Sharnoff. Lichens of North America. Yale University Press, 2001.

Brown, Deni. Enclyclopedia of Herbs and Their Uses. Reader's Digest Press, Que. 1995.
Bruneton, J Pharmacognosy, Phtyochemistry, Medicinal Plants, Lavoisier Pub. Paris, 1995
_____ Toxic Plants Dangerous to Humans and Animals. Editions TEC&Doc, Paris, '99.
Brunschwig, Hieronymus. Book of Distillation. Johnson Reprint Co No. 79. New York, 1971.
Bubar, Carol et al. Weeds of the Prairies. Alberta Agriculture Pub. Edmonton, 2000.
Buchanan, Carol. Brothers Crow, Sister Corn. Ten Speed Press, Berkeley, 1997.
Buckle, Jane. Clinical Aromatherapy. 2nd ed. Churchill Livingstone, Toronto, 2003.
Buhner, Stephen H. Sacred and Herbal Healing Beers, Siris Books, Boulder, Co, 1998
_____ Sacred Plant Medicine. Robert Rinehart, Boulder, Co. 1996.
_____ Herbal Antibiotics. Storey Books, Vermont, 1999.
_____ The Lost Language of Plants. Chelsea Green Pub. White River, Vt. 2002
_____ Secret Teachings of Plants. Bear & Co. Rochester, Vt. 2004.
_____ The Natural Testosterone Plan. Healing Arts Press, Rochester VT. 2007
Burbridge, Joan. Wildflowers of the Southern Interior of B.C. U. of B.C. Press, 1989.
Burger, W Flowers- How they changed the world. Prometheus Books. Amherst NY 2006.
Burgess, Isla. Weeds Heal. Viriditas Pub Group. Cambridge NZ 1998.
Burlando, Bruno et al, Herbal Principles in Cosmetics. CRC Press Boca Raton 2010.
Caius, Rev. Fr. Jean F., The Medicinal and Poisonous Plants of India, Scientific Pub, 1986.
Cameron, Elizabeth. A Floral ABC. John Wiley and Sons. Toronto. 1980.
Carpenter D. Snr Pub. Nursing Herbal Medicine Handbook, Springhouse Corp. 2001.
Carpinella, Maria et al. Novel Therapeutic Agents from Plants. Sci Pub. Enfield NJ 2009.
Carr, Emily. Wild Flowers. Royal BC Museum, Victoria, B.C, 2006
Carroll, Roisin. The Crane Bag Celtic Tree Ogam Oils , Feasibility Pub. Dublin
Carter, Bernard F. The Floral Birthday Book. Bloomsbury Books, London. 1990.
Casselman, Bill. Canadian Garden Words. Little, Brown & Co. Toronto, 1997.
Castleman, Michael. The Healing Herbs. Bantam Books. 1995.
Castro, Miranda. The Complete Homeopathy Handbook. MacMillan, 1990
Catty, Suzanne. Hydrosols the next Aromatherapy, Healing Arts Press, Vermont, 2001.
Cavers, Paul ed, The Biology of Canadian Weeds 62-83,Ag Institute of Canada, Ottawa, 1995
_____ 84-102 Ag Inst. of Canada, Ottawa, 2000.
_____ 103-129 Ag Inst. of Canada, Ottawa 2005
Ceres. Herbal Teas for Health and Healing. Healing Arts Press, Rochester, Vermont, 1984.
Chan, K, and Cheung L. Interactions between Chincese Herbal Medicinal Products and Orthodox Drugs. Harwood Academic Publishers, Canada, 2000.
Chandler, F. Herbs-Everyday Reference for Health Professionals, Can. Pharm Assoc. 2000
Chang & But. Pharmacology &Applications of Chinese Materia Medica, World Scientific, 86
Chang Chao-liang et al, Vegetables as Medicine, Pelanduk Pub, Malaysia, 1999.
Chappell, P. Emotional Healing with Homeopathy. North Atlantic Books. Berkeley, 2003.
Chase, Pamela & Pawlik, J. Newcastle Trees for Healing , Newcastle Pub. Van Nuys,1991
Chatroux, Sylvia Botanica Poetica. Poetica Press 2004 1-877-POETICA.
_____ Materica Poetica. Poetica Press 1998.
Chen, John K & Chen, Tina T. Chinese Medical Herbology & Pharmacology. Art of Medicine Press, City of Industry, CA 2004.
Chevalllier, Andrew. The Encyclopedia of Medicinal Plants. Reader's Digest, 1996.
Chishti, Hakim. The Traditional Healer, Healing Arts Press, Vermont,1988.
Clark, Ella E. Indian Legends of Canada. McClelland & Stewart. Toronto, 1960.
Coats, Peter. Flowers in History. Weidenfeld and Nicolson, London. 1970.
Coffey, Timothy.The History and Folklore of North American Wildflowers, Houghton-Mifflin, 1993.
Cohen, Kenneth. Honoring the Medicine. Random House, Toronto. 2003.

Conrad, Chris, Hemp for Health, Healing Arts Press, Rochester, Vermont, 1997.
Cook, Wm.H. The Physio-Medical Dispensatory. 1869. Reprinted by Eclectic Medical Publications, Portland, Oregon, 1985.
_____ A compendium of the new Materia medica together with additional descriptions of some old remedies. Wm. Cook Publisher, Chicago, 1896.
Cooper, J.C. Dictionary of Symbolic & Mythological Animals, Thorsons, London, 1992.
Cormack, R.G.H. Wild Flowers of Alberta. Hurtig Publishers, 1977
Coupland, Francois. The Encyclopedia of Edible Plants of N. America. Keats Pub. 1998.
Cousin, Pierre J. Eat Well, Be Well. Thorsons, London. 2001.
Cowan, Eliot. Plant Spirit Medicine. Swan Raven & Co. Box 726 Newberg, Oregon, 1995.
Cowan, Thomas. The Fourfold Path to Healing. New Trends Pub. Washington DC 2007.
Crane, Eva. Honey- A Comprhensive Survey , Heinemann Pub. London 1975.
Craydon D. & Bellows W. Floral Acupuncture. The Crossing Press Berkeley CA 2005.
Creekmore, H. Daffodils are Dangerous. Walker and Co. New York. 1966.
Crow, Tis Mal. Native Plants, Native Healing. Native Voices Book Pub. Box 99 Summertown, Tennessee, 2001 1-888-260-8458.
Crowell, Robert L. The Lore & Legends of Flowers. Thomas Crowell, New York, 1982.
Crowfoot & Baldensperger. From Cedar to Hyssop. Sheldon Press, London, 1932.
Cruden, Loren. Medicine Grove. Destiny Books. Inner Traditions Vermont. 1997.
Cummings, S. and Ullman, Dana. Everyone's Guide to Homeopathic Medicines, St. Martins Cupp, Melanie. Toxicology and Clinical Pharmacology of Herbal Products. Humana P. 1999
Curtin, LSM. Healing Herbs of the Upper Rio Grande. SouthWest Museum, Los Angeles 1965
Cutler & Cutler Eds. Biologically Active Natural Products: Agrochemicals, CRC Press 1999.
Dai Yin-fang&Liu Cheng-jun. Fruit As Medicine. Rams Skull Press, Kuranda, Aust. 1987
Dalton, David. Stars of the Meadow. Lindisfarne Books. Great Barrington, Mass. 2006.
D'Amelio Sr. Frank. Botanicals A Phytocosmetic Desk Reference CRC Press, Boca Raton, 99
Darby,Wm et al. Food: The Gift of Osiris, Vol 1. Academic Press, San Francisco, 1977
Darwin, Tess. The Scots Herbal, the Plant Lore of Scotland. Birlinn Ltd, Edinburgh 2008
Davidow, Joie. Infusions of Healing, A Treasury of Mexican-American Herbal Remedies, Fireside Books, New York, 1999.
Davis,W. El Gringo, New Mexico and Her People. Harpers, New York, 1857.
Demargaux, N. Phytotherapy. Herbal Health Publishers Ltd. 1989
De Bairacli Levy, Juliette. Herbal Handbook for Farm and Stable, Faber and Faber 1952
Deer Lame, J & Erdoes, R. Lame Deer Seeker of Visions. Washington Sq Press, 1976.
Deer, Thea Summer. Wisdom of the Plant Devas. Bear&Company Vermont 2011.
De Smet et al. Adverse Effects of Herbal Drugs. Springer-Verlag, Berlin. 1997.
Der Marderosian, Ara & Liberti L. Natural Product Medicine, George Stickley Co, Philadel.
Diederichsen, Axel. Coriander. Int. Plant Genetic Resources Institute. Rome, Italy. 1996.
DeRios, Marlene D. Hallucinogens: Cross Cultural Perspectives. U. New Mexico Press, 1984
DeSmet, P. et al. Adverse Effects of Herbal Drugs. vol 2 Springer-Verlag
Devi, Lila. The Essential Flower Essence Handbook. Crystal Clarity Pub. Nevada City 2007.
Dewey, Laurel. Plant Power- revised. Safe Goods/New Century Pub, Markham Ont, 2001.
Dewick, Paul M. Medicinal Natural Products.3rd Ed John Wiley and Sons, West Sussex, 2009.
Dixon, Bernard.Power Unseen, How Microbes Rule the World. W.H. Freeman, Oxford, 1994
Dow, Elaine. Simples and Worts. Historical Presentations, Topsfield, MA. 1982.
Duke, James. Handbook of Medicinal Herbs. CRC Press, Boca Raton, Florida, 1985
_____ Handbook of Edible Weeds. CRC Press. 1992
_____ The Green Pharmacy, Rodale Press, Emmaus, Pennsylvania, 1997.
_____ The Green Pharmacy Herbal Handbook, Rodale Press, 2000.

_____ Anti-aging Prescriptions. Rodale Press. 2001.
Dumas, Anne. Book of Plants and Symbols. English Ed. Octopus Pub. London 2004.
Dymock,Wm. Pharmacographia Indica, Vol 2, Kegan Paul, Trench, Trubner and Co. 1891
Earle, Liz. Vital Oils, Ebury Press, London, 1991.
Eason, Cassandra. Fabulous Creatures, Mythical Monsters… Greenwood Press, CT. 2008.
Eastman, John. The Book of Swamp and Bog... Stackpole Books, Mechanicsburg, Penn, 1995
Ebadi, M. Pharmacodynamic Basis of Herbal Medicine, CRC Press, Boca Raton. 2002.
Eckey, E.W. Vegetable Fats and Oils, Rheingold Publishing Co, New York, 1954.
Eclare, Melanie. Flower Spirit Cards. Quadrille Publishing, London, England, 2004.
Edwards, Lawrence. The Vortex of Life. Floris Books. Edinburgh 2nd Ed. 2006.
Eisner T et al. Secret Weapons. Belknap Press, Harvard U Press. Cambridge & London 2005.
Ellingwood F. American Materia Medica, Eclectic Med. Pub. Portand, Oregon, reprint, 1983
Elliot, Douglas B. Roots . Chatham Press, Old Greenwich Conneticut.
Ellis, Hattie. Sweetness & Light. Hodder and Stoughton, London, 2004.
Erdoes & Ortiz. American Indian Myths and Legends, Pantethon Books, New York, 1984.
Erichsen-Brown,Charlotte. Use of Plants for the Past 500 Years, Breezy Creeks Press, 1979
_____ Medicinal and Other Uses of North American Plants, General Pub, 1979.
Erickson, David, Wai Kit Nip Food uses of whole oil and protein seeds, Amer. Oil Chemists Society, 1989.
Eskin, N. A. Michael, Tamir, S. Dictionary of Nutraceuticals and Functional Foods. CRC Press, 2006.
Etkin, Nina. Edible Medicines, An Ethnopharmacology of Food. U Arizona Press. 2006.
Evans, W.C. Trease and Evans' Pharmacognosy. WB Saunders Co. Toronto, 2000.
Fang Jing Pei, Dr. Natural Remedies from the Chinese Cupboard. Weatherhill, 1998.
Farmer-Knowles,Helen. The Healing Garden. Sterling Publishing, New York, 1998.
Fielder, Mildred. Plant Medicne and Folklore, Winchester Press, New York, 1975.
Felter, Harvery and Lloyd, John. King's American Dispensatory . 1898.
Reprinted by Eclectic Medical Publications, Portland Oregon, 1983.
Ferguson, Gary. Spirits of the Wild. Clarkson Potter/Random New York, 1996.
Fernie, W.T. Dr. Old Fashioned Herbal Remedies. Coles Pub. Toronto, 1980. Reprint.
Fingerman M. et al editors. Bioremediation of Aquatic and Terresrial Ecosytems. Sci Pub. Enfield NH 2005.
Fischer-Rizzi, S. Complete Aromatherapy Handbook, Sterling Pub. New York. 1990.
_____ The Complete Incense Book, Sterling Pub. New York 1998.
_____ Medicine of the Earth, Rudra Press, Portland, Oregon, 1996
Florey, H.W. et al. Antibiotics vol 1. Oxford University Press. London 1949.
Ford, Gillian. Plant Names Explained. Friends of the Devonian Botanic Garden, #16, 1984
Foster, Steven. Herbal Renaissance, Gibbs Smith Pub. Salt Lake City
_____ & Yue Chongxi. Herbal Emissaries, Healing Arts Press, Vermont, 1992
_____ & Johnson R. Desk Reference to Nature's Medicine. Nat Geographic. Washington, D.C.
Fox, H. M. Gardening with Herbs. Macmillan Pub. New York 1933.
Freeman, D. & Mongeau D. Nettles and More… Vol One. Self published 2nd printing 2009.
Freeman, Lyn. Mosby's Complementary & Alternative Medicine.3rd Ed. Mosby Elsevier 2009
Friedman, Sara Ann, Celebrating the Wild Mushroom, Dodd, Mead & Co. New York, 1986
Friend, Tim. The Third Domain: the Untold Story of Archaea. Joseph Henry Press. 2007.
Fugh-Berman, Adriane. The 5-minute Herb &Dietary Supplement Consult. Lippincott Williams &Wilkins, Philadelphia 2003.
Gaertner, Erika. Reap without Sowing. General Store Publishing, Burnstown, Ont. 1995
Galun, Margalith. Handbook of Lichenology, CRC Press, 1988

Garran, Thomas. Western herbs according to Traditional Chinese Medicine. Healing Arts Press. 2008.
Garrett, J.T. The Cherokee Herbal. Bear&Company, Rochester, Vermont. 2003.
Genders, Roy. Floral Scents of the World . St. Martin's Press, London, 1977
Geuter, Herbs in Nutrition. Bio-Dynamic Agricultural Assoc. London. 1978.
Gildemeister, E. The Volatile Oils. John Wiley and Sons, New York. 1916
Gifford, Jane. The Wisdom of Trees. Sterling Pub. New York 2000.
Gill S. & Sullivan I. Dictionary of Native American Mythology. Oxford U Press 1992.
Gilmore, M.R. Uses of Plants by Indians of the Missouri river region. 33rd Annual Report Bureau American Ethnology, 1911-12, Washington D.C. 1919.
Gladstar R & Hirsch P. Planting the Future. Healing Arts Press, Rochester, Vt. 2000.
Gladstar, Rosemary. Family Herbal. Storey Books, North Adams, Mass. 2001.
Glasby, J.S. Dictionary of Plants Containing Secondary Metabolites, Taylor & Francis, London 1991.
Godfrey, A & Saunders P. Principles and Practices of Naturopathic Botanical Medicine, Vol 1, CCNM Press Toronto ON 2010.
Goodrick-Clarke, Clare. Alchemical Medicine for the 21st Century. Healing Arts Press. 2010.
Gordon, David G. The Compleat Cockroach. Ten Speed Press, Berkeley, CA. 1996.
Gordon, Lesley. The Mystery and Magic of Trees & Flowers. Grange Books. London 1993.
Gottesfeld, Leslie M. Johnson. Plants, Land and People, A Study of Wet'suwet'en Ethnobotany.U of A, 1993.
Grae, Ida. Nature's Colors, Dyes From Plants. Macmillan Pub. New York, 1974.
Graham, Frances K. Plant lore of an Alaskan Island. Alaska Northwest Pub. 1985
Grange, Michael etal, Handbook of Plants with Pest Control Properties, J. Wiley& Son 1988
Gray, Bev. The Boreal Herbal. Wild Food & Medicine Plants of the North. Aroma Borealis Press 2011
Green, James. The Male Herbal . Crossing Press, Freedom, California, 1991.
_____ The Herbal Medicine-Maker's Handbook. Crossing Press, Freedom CA 2000
Green, Jonathan. Consuming Passions. Sphere Books, London, 1985.
Grey Wolf. Earth Signs, Raincoast Books, Vancouver, B.C. 1998.
Grieve, M. A Modern Herbal. Jonathan Cape. 1931
Griffiths, Deirdre. Elk Island National Park. U. of Alberta Press, 1979.
Grigson, Geoffrey. A Herbal of All Sorts. Phoenix House, London
Grimaud, Baptiste,Paul. TAROT DES FLEURS, France Cartes, France 1989
Grimshaw, John. The Gardener's Atlas. Firefly Books, Willowdale, Ont. 2002.
Grohmann,Gerbert. The Plant Vol 2, Bio-Dynamic Farming & Gardening Assoc. 1989.
Gruenwald et al, Ed. PDR for Herbal Medicines. 4th Ed. Thomson Pub. 2007.
Guillet, Alma. Make Friends of Trees and Shrubs. Doubleday & Co. New York, 1962.
Gumbel, Dietrich. Principles of Holistic Skin Therapy with Herb Essences. Haug Pub. Heidelberg 1986.
Gurudas. The Spiritual Properties of Herbs , Cassandra Press, 1988
_____ Flower Essences and Vibrational Healing, Cassandra Press, 1983
Hageneder, Fred. The Spirit of Trees. Continuum. NY and London. 2005.
Hale, Mason. The Biology of Lichens. Edward Arnold Pub. London, 1967.
Hall, Dorothy. Creating Your Herbal Profile , Keats, 1988
Hallworth, B & Chinnappa CC. Plants of the Kananaskis Country U of A Press 1997.
Hanchuk, Rena. The Word and Wax. Can Inst of Ukrainian Studies Press, Edmonton, 1999.
Hanson, J, & Morrison D. Of Kinkajous, Capybaras, Horned Beetles...Harper Collins, NY '91
Harbourne & Baxter. The Handbook of Natural Flavonoids Vol 1&2. John Wiley & Sons, 1999
_____ Phytochemical Dictionary. Taylor & Francis 1993.

Harrington, Geri. Growing Your Own Chinese Vegetables, MacMillan, N.Y. 1978.
Harrington, H.D. Edible Native Plants of the Rocky Mtns. U. of New Mexico Press, 1967.
Harris, Ben C. Eat the Weeds, Keats Pub. New Cannan, Conneticut 1973.
_____ Make Use of Your Garden Plants. General Pub. New York. 1978.
Harris, Marjorie. Botanica North America. Harper Collins, New York, 2003.
Harrison, Nora. Flower Remedy Rhymes , self published, England, 1990.
Hart, Jeff. Montana Native Plants and Early Peoples, Montana Historical Society Press. '92
_____ The Ethnobotany of the Northern Cheyenne Indians of Montana. Journal of Ethnopharmacology 1981 4.
Hartung, Tammi. Growing 101 Herbs That Heal. Storey Books, Pownal, Vt. 2000.
Hartwell, Jonathan, Plants Used Against Cancer. Quarterman Pub. 1982
Hartzell, Jr. H. The Yew Tree A Thousand Whispers. Hulogosi, Box 1188, Eugene, OR 1991.
Harvey, C & Cochrane A. The Healing Spirit of Plants. Godsfield Press, Sterling Pr N.Y. 1999
Harvey Clare. The New Encyclopedia of Flower Remedies. Watkins Pub. London 2007.
Hatfield, Gabrielle. Encyclopedia of Folk Medicine. ABC CLIO Santa Barbara. 2004.
Haughton, Claire. Green Immigrants. Harcourt Brace Jovanovich. New York and London.
Hawksworth, Frank & Wiens, D. Dwarf Mistletoes, Ag Handbook 709, USDA, Wash, DC, '96
Health Canada, Native Foods and Nutrition. Medical Services Branch, 1995.
Heatherington, M. and Steck,W. Natural Chemicals from Northern Prairie Plants, Ag West Biotech Publishers, Saskatoon, Canada. 1997.
Heilmeyer, Marina. The Language of Flowers-Symbols & Myths. Prestel Pub. Munich 2001.
Heinerman, John. Encyclopedia of Nuts, Berries and Seeds, Parker Publishing, 1995.
_____ Encyclopedia of Healing Herbs & Spices. Parker Pub. N.Y. 1996.
Heinrich, Bernd. Winter World The Ingenuity of animal survival. HarperCollins. NY 2003.
Heinrich, Clark. Magic Mushrooms in Religion and Alchemy. Park St. Press, VT. 2002.
Heiser, Charles B. Jr. Of Plants and People. U. of Oklahoma Press, 1985.
Hellson, John C, Ethnobotany of the Blackfoot Indians No. 19, National Museums of Canada, Ottawa 1974.
Henderson, Robert K. The Neighborhood Forager. Key Porter Books, Toronto, 2000.
Hendrickson, Robert. Encycl of Word and Phrase Origins. Facts on File Inc. NewYork, 1997.
Hendry, G. Natural Food Colorants , Blackie and Son, Glasgow Scotland, 1992.
Henry, J. David. Canada's Boreal Forest. Smithsonian Institute 2002.
Hilarion. Wildflowers, Their Occult Gifts. Marcus Books, Queensville, Ont. 1982.
Hobbs, Christopher. Usnea . The Herbal Antibiotic. Botanica Press 1986.
_____ Medicinal Mushrooms, Botanica Press, Santa Cruz, 1995.
Hoffman, David The Holistic Herbal. Findhorn Press, 1983.
_____ Welsh Herbal Medicine. Abercastle Publications, Dyfed, 1978.
_____ Medical Herbalism. Healing Arts Press, Rochester, VT, 2003.
Hole, Lois. Favorite Trees and Shrubs. Lone Pine Pub. Edmonton Alta. 1997.
_____ Perennial Favorites. Lone Pine Pub. 1995.
Holm, LeRoy G. World Weeds, John Wiley and Sons, 1997.
Holmes, Peter. The Energetics of Western Herbs, Vol 1 and 2, Artemis Press, 1989.
_____ Jade Remedies, Vol 1 and 2, Snow Lotus Press, Boulder 1996.
Hopman, Ellen. A Druid's Herbal, Destiny Books, Rochester, Vermont. 1995.
Howarth, D& Kahlee Keane. Wild Medicines of the Prairies Self Published, 1995.
_____ Native Medecines Self Published , 1995
Hozeski, Bruce. Hildegard's Healing Plants. Beacon Press. Boston, Mass. 2001.
Hsu, Hong-Yen. Oriental Materia Medica, Keats Publishing,Connecticut, 1986.
Huang, Kee Chang. The Pharmacolocy of Chinese Herbs. 2nd Edition, CRC Press, 1999.
Hu-Nan. A Barefoot Doctor's Manual. Running Press, Philadelphia, 1977.

Hudson, James B. Antiviral Compounds from Plants, CRC Press, Florida, 1990
Hudson, Rick. A Field Guide to Gold, Gemstone and Mineral Sites. Orca Pub, Victoria, 1999
Hurley, Judith. The Good Herb Wm. Morrow and Co. New York, 1995.
Hutchens, Alma. Indian Herbology of North America. Merco. 1969
Ingram, Cass. Supermarket Remedies. Knowledge House, Buffalo Grove, Ill. 1998.
Inkpen W & Van Eyk, R. Guide to the Common Native Trees and Shrubs of Alberta, Government of Alberta, Environmental Protection, 1995.
James & Keeler, Poisonous Plants- 3rd Int. Symposium, Iowa State U. Press, 1992.
Jason, Dan & Nancy. Some Useful Wild Plants, Talon Books, Vancouver, 1972.
Jiao Shu-De. Ten Lectures on the Use of Medicinals. Paradigm Pub. Brookline, Mass. 2003.
Johnson, Kershaw, MacKinnon & Pojar Plants of the Western Boreal Forest and Aspen Parkland, Lone Pine Press, Edmonton, Alberta 1995.
Johnson, L. Tending the Earth A Gardener's Manifesto. Penguin Books, Toronto, 2002.
Johnson, Leslie. Journal of Ethnobotany and Ethnomedicine. 2006 2:29.
_____ Health, Wholeness & the Land: Gitksan Traditional Plant Use and Healing. U of Alberta 1997.
Jones, Alison. Larousse Dictionary of World Folklore. Larousse, New York, 1995.
Jones, Pamela. Just Weed, History, Myths and Uses. Prentice Hall Press, Toronto, 1991.
Kamm, Minnie W. Old Time Herbs for Northern Gardens Little Brown & Co. 1938.
Kane, Charles W. Herbal Medicine of the American Southwest. Lincoln Town Press. 2007.
_____ Herbal Medicine: trends and traditions. Lincoln Town Press 2009.
Kapoor, L.D. CRC Handbook of Ayurvedic Medicinal Plants, CRC Press, Boca Raton, 1990.
Kari, Priscilla. Tanaina Plantlore. National Park Service, Alaska Region 1987.
Kaur, Sat Dharam. The Complete Natural Medicine Guide to Breast Cancer. Robert Rose Inc Toronto, 2003.
Kavash E, Barrie & Barr K, American Indian Healing Arts. Bantam Books, Toronto 1999.
_____ The Medicine Wheel Garden. Bantam Books, N.Y. 2002.
Kay, Margarita Artschwager. Healing with Plants in the American and Mexican West, The University of Arizona Press, Tucson. 1996
Kays, S & Nottingham S. Biology and Chemistry of Jerusalem Artichoke. CRC Press 2008.
Keane, Kahlee & Howarth,D. The Standing People. Saskatoon, Saskatchewan. 2003.
Kee Chang Huang, The Pharmacology of Chinese Herbs, 2nd Edition, CRC Press, 1999.
Kemp, Cynthia. Cactus and Company. Desert Alchemy, Tucson, Arizona, 1993.
Kenner D &Requena Y. Botanical Medicine: .Paradigm Pub. Brookline, Mass, 1996.
Kerik, Joan. Living with the Land:Use of Plants by the Native People of Alberta, Alberta Culture, Circulating Exhibits Program, National Museums of Canada Fund, 1981.
Kershaw, Linda. Edible & Medicinal Plants of the Rockies, Lone Pine, Edmonton 2000.
_____ Alberta Wayside Wildflowers. Lone Pine, Edmonton, 2003.
_____ Saskatchewan Wayside Wildflowers. Lone Pine, Edmonton, 2003.
_____ Manitoba Wayside Wildflowers. Lone Pine, Edmonton, 2003.
Kershaw, L. et al. Rare Vascular Plants of Alberta. U. of Alberta Press, Edmonton, 2001.
Kershaw, MacKinnon & Pojar. Plants of the Rocky Mountains. Lone Pine, Edmonton 1998.
Keys, John. D. Chinese Herbs, Charles E. Tuttle Co. 1976.
Kimmerer,Robin. Gathering Moss. Oregon State University Press, Corvallis, 2003.
Kindscher, Kelly. Medicnal Wild Plants of the Prairies. Univ. Press of Kansas. 1987.
King, Francis X. Rudolf Steiner and Holistic Medicine. Rider & Co. England, 1986.
Klein, Carol. Plant Personalities. Timber Press, Portland, Oregon. 2005.
Klein, Richard. The Green World. 2nd edition. Harper Collins, 1987.
Kloss, Jethro. Back to Eden. Woodbridge Press Pub.Co. Santa Barbara, Ca. 1975.
Knab, Sophie H. Polish Herbs, Flowers and Folk Medicine. Hippocrene Books, N.Y. 1999.

Knowles, Hugh. Woody Ornamentals for the Prairies. U. of Alberta , 1995.
Knudtson,P & Suzuki D. Wisdom of the Elders. Greystone Books. Vancouver BC 2006.
Kraft, K & Hobbs C. Pocket Guide to Herbal Medicine. Thieme, N.Y. 2004.
Kranich, Ernst M. Planetary Influences Upon Plants. Bio-Dynamic Lit. Wyoming RI 1984.
Krymow, V. Healing Plants of the Bible. Wild Goose Pub. Glasgow, UK 2002.
Kuhnlein, Harriet and Turner, Nancy. Traditional Plant Foods of Canadian Indigenous Peoples. Gordon and Breach Science Publishers. 1991.
Kuijt, Job. The Biology of Parasitic Flowering Plants, U. of California Press, 1969
Kunkele, U. & Lohmeyer, T. Herbs for Healthy Living. Parragon Pub. Bath UK 2007.
Lacey, Laurie. Micmac Medicines Remedies and Recollections. Nimbus Pub. Halifax, 1993.
Lahring, Heinjo. Water and Wetland Plants of the Prairie Provinces, Can Plains Research Center, U. of Regina, 2003
Lambert, Grant. Falling Leaf Essences. Healing Arts Press, Rochester Vermont, 2002.
Lamont, SM. The Fisherman Lake Slave and their environment: a story of floral and faunal resources. Master's thesis. U. of Saskatchewan, Saskatoon, 1977.
Langenheim, Jean. Medicinal Plant Resins. Timber Press Portland Oregon 2003.
Larsen,Henning. An Old Icelandic Medical Miscellany, Norske Akademi, Oslo, Norway '31
Lavabre, Marcel. Aromatherapy Workbook. Healing Arts Press, Vermont. 1990.
Lawless, Julia, The Encyclopedia of Essential Oils , Element Books, 1992.
LeClaire,N &Cardinal,G. Alberta Elders' Cree Dictionary, U of Alberta Press, 1998.
Leduc, M.A. The Explorers Guide to Boreal Forest Plants, Hwy Book Shop, Cobalt, Ont. 1997
Leighton, Anna L. Wild Plant Use by the Woods Cree (NIHITHAWAK) of East-Central Saskatchewan . Paper no. 101, National Museums of Canada, Ottawa, 1985
Lepore, Donald. The Ultimate Healing System. Woodland Books, Provo, Utah, 1988.
Le Strange, Richard, A History of Herbal Plants. Arco Pub. New York. 1977.
Leung, Albert. Chinese Herbal Remedies. Universe Books, New York, 1984.
Leung & Foster, Encyclopedia of Common Natural Ingredients, J. Wiley&Sons, N.Y. 1996.
Levey,M. The Medical Formulary or Aqrabadhin of Al-Kindi U of Wisconsin Press, 1966
Leyel, C.F. Elixirs of Life, Faber and Faber, London.1948
Li, Thomas. Medicinal Plants, Culture, Utilization & Phytopharmacology. Technomic Publishing, Lancaster, Pennsylvania, 2000.
Li, Thomas. Chinese and related North American Herbs. CRC Press, Boca Raton, 2002.
Libster, Martha. Delmar's Integrative Herb Guide for Nurses. Delmar, 2002.
Lininger et al. The Natural Pharmacy. Healthnotes, Prima Pub. Rocklin Ca, 1999.
L'Orange Darlena, Herbal Healing Secrets of the Orient. Prentice Hall, New Jersey, 1998.
Lock, Carolyn. Country Colours. Nova Scotia Museum. 1981
Lovejoy, Sharon. Sunflower Houses. Workman Pub Co. New York 2001.
Lu, Henry. Using Foods to Stay Young, Sterling Press, New York, 1996.
_____ Chinese Natural Cures. Black Dog & Leventhal Pub. New York, 1994
Luetjohann, Sylvia. The Healing Power of Black Cumin. Lotus Light, Twin Lakes, WI, 1998
Lyle, Katie Letcher. The Wild Berry Book, NorthWord Press, Minocqua, WI, 1994.
Mabey, Richard. Plantcraft. Universe Books. 1978.
MacKinnon, Pojar, Coupe. Plants of Northern British Columbia. Lone Pine Press, 1992.
Mailhebiau, Philippe. Portraits in Oils. C.W. Daniel Company, Essex, England, 1995.
Malmud, René. The Amazon Problem, trans by M. Stein, Spring Pub. Dallas TX, 1980.
Maloof, Joan. Teaching the Trees, Lessons from the Forest. U Georgia Pr, Athena GA. 2005.
Manandhar, N.P. Plants and People of Nepal. Timber Press, Portland, Oregon, 2002.
Maple, Eric. The Secret Lore of Plants and Flowers. Robert Hale Ltd. London 1980.
March, Kathryn & Andrew. The Wild Plant Companion. Meridian Hill Pub. 1986.
Marles, Robin. The Ethnobotany of the Chipewyan of Northern Saskatchewan, 1984. Thesis.

_________ et al. Aboriginal Plant Use in Canada's Northwest Boreal Forest. UBC Press, Vancouver, and Natural Resources Canada, 2000
McBride, L.R. Practical Folk Medicine of Hawaii. Petroglyph Press, Hilo,Hawaii, 1975.
McCune B. & Geiser L. Macrolichens of the Pacific Northwest. Oregon State U. Press, 1997
McFarland, Phoenix. The Complete Book of Magical Names. Llewellyn Pub. St Paul 1996
McGrath, Judy. Dyes from Lichens and Plants. Van Nostrand Rheinhold, 1977.
McGuffin, Nancy. Spectrum: dye plants of Ontario. Burr House Spinner, Richmond Hill '86
McIntyre, Anne. The Complete Woman's Herbal, Henry Holt, New York, 1995.
Mears, R & Hillman,G. Wild Food. Hodder and Stoughton
MELODY. Love is in the Earth, A Kaleidoscope of Crystals. Earth Love Pub. Col. 1995.
Mercatante, A. S. The Facts on File Encyclopedia of World Mythology. New York 1988
Merriam, C. Hart. Dawn of the World, Weird Tales of Mewan Indians. Arthur H. Clark, Cleveland, 1910
Meyer, George et al. Folk Medicine and Herbal Healing, Charles Thomas, Springfield, 1981
Meyerowitz,Steve. Sprout It! The Sprout House, Box 1100,Great Barrington, MA, 1993.
Meyers, Edward C. Basic Bush Survival, Hancock House, Surrey, B.C. 1997.
Miller, L &Murray,W. Herbal Medicinals A Clinician's Guide. Hawthorn Press, N.Y. 1998.
Miller, Sandra. Editor Echinacea- Medicinal and Aromatic Plants. CRC Press, 2004.
Mills S. & Bone,K. Principles and Practice of Phytotherapy. Churchill Livingstone, 2000.
_____ The Essential Guide to Herbal Safety. Churchill Livingstone, 2005.
Mills, Simon. Out of the Earth. Viking Penquin Books, Toronto. 1991.
Millsbaugh, Charles. American Medicinal Plants, Dover Pub. New York, 1974
Milne, Courtney. Visions of the Goddess, Penguin Studio, Toronto, 1998
Minnis & Elisens. Biodiversity and Native America. U. Oklahoma Press, 2000.
Mitchel, Jr. Wm. Plant Medicine in Practice. Churchill Livingstone, St. Louis, 2003.
Moerman, Daniel, Medicinal Plants of Native America. U of Michigan No. 19, 1986
Mohammed, G. Catnip & Kerosene Grass Candlenut Books, Sault Ste. Marie, Ont, 2002.
Montgomery, Pam. Plant Spirit Healing. Bear and Company, Rochester, VT 2008.
Moore, Michael. Los Remedios. Red Crane Books, 1990
_____ Medicinal Plants of the Desert and Canyon West. Museum of New Mexico Press 1989
_____ Medicinal Plants of the Mountain West, Museum of New Mexico Press '79
_____ Med Plants of the Mountain West. Revised, expanded. 2003
_____ Medicinal Plants of the Pacific West, Red Crane Books, 1993
More, Daphne. The Bee Book, Universe Books, New York, 1976.
Morelli, I. et al. Selected Medicinal Plants. University of Pisa. FAO 53/1
Morton, Julia. Major Medicinal Plants . Charles Thomas, Springfield, Illinois 1977
_____ Atlas of Medicinal Plants of Middle America, Bahamas to Yucatan. 1981
Moss, E.H. Flora of Alberta. University of Toronto Press. 1983
Mother, The. Flowers and their Messages. Sri Aurobindo Ashram Trust, India 1979.
Mourning Dove. Coyote Stories. Caxton Press Caldwell Idaho. 1933.
Mowrey, Daniel. The Scientific Validation of Herbal Medicine. Cormorant Books, 1986.
Mucz, Michael. Baba's Kitchen Medicines. U of Alberta Press, Edmonton, 2012.
Mulders, Evelyn. Western Herbs for Eastern Meridian & 5 Element Theory. Self publ. 2006.
Mulligan, G editor The biology of Canadian Weeds, 1-32 Pub. 1693 Ag Canada 1979
_____ 33-61 Pub. 1765 Ag Canada 1984
Murphy, Cristine Editor, Practical Home Care Medicine, Lantern Books, New York, 2001
Murray, Michael. The Pill Book Guide to Natural Medicines. Bantam Books, April, 2002.
_____ & Pizzorno, J. The condensed Encycl of Healing Foods. Pocket Books NY 2005.
Naegele, Thomas A. Edible and Medicinal Plants of the Great Lakes Region, Wilderness Adventure Books, Davisburg, Michigan. 1996.

Naiman, Ingrid. Cancer Salves, A Botanical Approach to Treatment. N. Atlantic Books, 99.
Nesse R & Williams G. Why We Get Sick. Vintage Books/Random House, New York, 1996.
Neuwinger H.D. African Traditional Medicine. Medpharm Sci. Pub. Stuttgart 2000.
_____ African Ethnobotany, Poisons and Drugs. Chapman & Hall, London 1996.
Newcombe C.F. unpub notes on Haida plants. Dept of Anthro. Am Mus Nat Hist. NY 1897
_____ unpublished papers. Prov Archives B.C. Victoria. 1898-1913.
Nicander. The Poems and Poetical Fragments. Cambridge U. Press, New York, 1953.
Norman,Howard. Northern Tales. Pantheon Books, New York, 1990.
Northcote, Rosalind. The Book of Herbs. John Lane: The Bodley Head, London, 1912.
Null, Gary. The Clinician's Handbook of Natural Healing. Kensington Books, N.Y. 1997.
Olive, Barbara. The Flower Healer. Cico Books, London and New York. 2007.
Ollsin, Don. Herbal Healing Journey-Playful Workbook. Aquiline Comm, Victoria,BC 1998.
Ootoova I. et al. Interviewing Inuit Elders, Perspectives on Traditional Health. Vol 5, Nunavut Arctic College, Box 600, Iqaluit, Nunavut X0Z 0H0.
Page, George. Inside the Animal Mind. Doubleday, New York, 1999.
Pallasdowney, Rhonda. The Complete Book of Flower Essences. New World Library, 2002.
Pappalardo, Joe. Sunflowers (the secret history). The Overlook Press. Woodstock NY 2008.
Parish, Coupé & Lloyd. Plants of S. Interior British Columbia. Lone Pine Edmonton 1996
Park, Willard Z. Ethnographic Notes on the Norhern Paiute of Western Nevada, 1933-40 compiled by Catherine Fowler, U. of Utah, Salt Lake City, 1989.
Parvati, J. Hygieia, A Woman's Herbal. Freestone Collective. 1978
Paturi, Felix Nature, Mother of Invention. Harper and Row Pub. New York. 1976.
Peirce,Andrea. Practical Guide to Natural Medicines. Stonesong Press. 1999.
Pelikan, W. Healing Plants. Mercury Press, Spring Valley NY 1997.
Pellowski, Anne. Hidden Stories in Plants. MacMillan Pub. New York. 1990.
Penoel,Daniel & Franchomme, P. L'Aromatherapie Exactement , Roger Jollois, France, 1990
Peneol, Daniel. Medecine Aromatique, Medecine Planetaire. Roger Jollois France 1991.
_____ & Peneol, Rose-Marie. Natural Home Health Care Using Essential Oils. Osmobiose Pub. 1998.
People of 'Ksan, The. Gathering What the Great Nature Provided. Douglas & McIntyre. Vancouver, B.C. 1980.
Peters, Josephine & Ortiz B, After the First Full Moon in April. Left Coast Press. Walnut Creek CA, 2010.
Pettitt,Sabina. Energy Medicine, Healing from the Kingdoms of Nature, Pacific Essences, Box 8317, Victoria, B.C. V8W 3R9 Canada, 1999
Phaneuf, Holly. Herbs Demystified. Marlowe and Company, New York. 2005
Pielou, E.C. The Naturalist's Guide to the Arctic. U. of Chicago Press. 1994.
Pieroni, A & Price L. Eating and Healing, Trad Food as Medicine. Haworth Press. N.Y. 2006.
Pfeiffer E. The Earth's Face and Human Destiny, Rodale Press, Emmaus, Pa. 1947.
Plotkin, Mark. Medicine Quest. Viking Penguin Books, New York, 2000.
Pojar, J & MacKinnon, A. Plants of Coastal British Columbia Lone Pine Edmonton 1994.
Pollock, L. With Faith and Physic: the life of a tudor gentlewoman. Collins & Brown,1993.
Polya, Gideon. Biochemical Targets of Plant Bioactive Comp. CRC Press, Boca Raton 2003
Pond, Barbara, A Sampler of Wayside Herbs, Chatham Press, Riverside, Conn.
Pressor, Arthur, Pharmacist's Guide to Medicinal Herbs, Smart Pub. Petaluma, CA,2000
Price, Len & Shirley. Understanding Hydrolats. Churchill Livingstone, Toronto, 2004.
_____ Aromatherapy for Health Professionals. Churchill Livingstone 1995.
Purvis, William. Lichens. Smithsonian Institution Press. Washington D.C. 2000
Quin, Frederick F. The Flora Homoeopathica. B. Jain Pub. New Delhi, India. 1997.
Radin, Paul. The Winnebago Tribe, Bur of Am Ethnology, Smithsonian Inst. 37th. 1923.

Rätsch, C. Plants of Love, The History of Aphrodisiacs. Ten Speed Press, Berkeley,1997.
_____ The Dictionary of Sacred & Magical Plants. ABC-CLIO St Barbara 1992.
_____ The Encyclopedia of Psychoactive Plants. Park St Press. 2005.
Reaume, Tom. 620 Wild Plants of North America. Nature Manitoba. Canadian Plains Research Center, U of Regina, U of Toronto Press. 2009.
Reckeweg, Hans-Heinrich, Materia Medica, Vol 1. Aurelia-Verlag GmbH, Baden Baden 1996.
Reich, Lee. Uncommon Fruits Worthy of Attention, Addison-Wesley Pub. 1991.
Reid, Daniel, A handbook of Chinese Healing Herbs, Shambala, Boston, 1995
Rhode, David. Native Plants of Southern Nevada. U of Utah Press. 2002.
Richards B & Kanecko A. Japanese Plants- Know Them &Use Them. Shufunotomo, Tokyo 1995
Richardson, David. The Vanishing Lichens. David and Charles, Vancouver, BC, 1975
Riddle, John M. Eve's Herbs. Harvard U Press. Cambridge Mass. 1997.
_____ Goddesses, Elixirs and Witches. Palgrave MacMillan. England 2010.
Rister, Robert. Healing Without Medication. Basic Health Pub. N. Bergen, N.J. 2003.
Roberts, Jonathan. The Origins of Fruit and Vegetables. Universe Pub. New York. 2001.
Robicsek, F. The Smoking God: Tobacco....Norman: U. of Oklahoma Press, 1978.
Robinson, Peggy. Profiles of Northwest Plants. Far West Book Service. Portland, OR 1979
Rogers, Dilwyn. Edible, Medicinal, Useful & Poisonous Wild Plants of the Northern Great Plains —South Dakota Region. Buechel Memorial Lakota Museum, St. Francis,SD, 1980.
Rogers, Pattiann. Firekeeper:New & Selected Poems. Milkweed Editions, 1994.
Rogers, Robert Dale. Sundew Moonwort Vols-1-7, self-published. Edmonton 1995-present.
_____ Rogers' Herbal Manual. Karamat Wilderness Ways, Edmonton, 2000.
_____ & Capital Health, Herbal Drug Interactions. Mediscript Comm. 2003.
_____ The Fungal Pharmacy, The Complete Guide to Medicinal Mushrooms and Lichens of North America, North Atlantic Books 2011.
Rombi, Max. Phytotherapy. Herbal Health Publishers. U.K. 1990.
Rosengarten,Jr. F. The Book of Edible Nuts. Walker and Co. New York. 1984.
Ross, Gary. Nature's Guide to Healing. Freedom Press, Topanga, Ca. 2000.
Ross, Ivan. Medicinal Plants of the World. Vol 1 Humana Press, Totowa, New Jersey. 1999.
_____ Vol 2 Humana Press, Totowa, N. J. 2002.
Rotella, Rev. Alexis. The Essence of Flowers, Jade Mountain Press, N.J. 1991.
Royer F. & Dickinson R. Plants of Alberta. Lone Pine Pub. Edmonton, AB. 2007.
Rudginsky, Marlene The Flower Speaks. U.S. Games Systems, Stamford, Conn. 1999.
Rupp, Rebecca. Red Oaks and Black Birches , Storey Comm. Garden Way Publishing. 1990
Russell, Sharman Apt. Anatomy of a Rose. Perseus Pub. Cambridge, Mass. 2001.
_____ An Obsession with Butterflies. Perseus Publishing 2003.
Ryan, J et al, Traditional Dene Medicine. Lac La Martre NWT, 1993.
Ryden, Hope. Wildflowers around the year. Clarion Books, New York. 2001.
Ryrie, Charlie. Garden Folklore That Works. Reader's Digest. Pleasantville, NY 2001.
Sagadic O. & Ozcan M. Food Control 2003 14.
Salmon, Wm. Botanologia: The English Herbal. London: I. Dawkes, 1710.
Sandberg & Corrigan. Natural Remedies, their origins and uses. Taylor & Francis 2001.
Sanders, Jack. The Secrets of Wildflowers. The Lyons Press, Guilford, CT, 2003.
Sapolsky, Robert. The Trouble with Testosterone. Scribner, New York. 1997.
Sauer, Johann Christopher, Compendious Herbal-see Weaver below.
Savage, Candace. Bees, Nature's Little Wonders. Greystone Books. Vancouver 2008.
Schalkwijk-Barendsen, Helene. Mushrooms of Western Canada . Lone Pine Pub. 1991.
Schar, Douglas. The Backyard Medicine Chest. Elliott&Clark Pub. Washington, DC. 1995.

Scheffer, Mechthild, Bach Flower Therapy, Theory and Practice, Healing Arts Press, 1988
Schenk, George. Moss Gardening. Timber Press, Portland Oregon. 1997.
Schnaubelt, Kurt. Medical Aromatherapy. Frog Ltd. Berkeley CA. 1999.
Schneider, Anny. Wild Medicinal Plants. Key Porter Books, Toronto. 2002.
Schnell, Donald. Carnivorous Plants. 2nd Ed. Timber Press, Portland, Oregon, 2002.
Schofield, Janice. Discovering Wild Plants. Alaska Northwest Books. 1989.
_____ Nettles. Keats Publishing, New Canaan, Conneticut, 1998.
Schulman, Robert. Solve It With Supplements. Rodale Press. New York. 2007.
Shapiro, R & Rapkins J. Awakening to the Plant Kingdom, Cassandra Press 1991.
Shauenberg, Paul and Paris. Guide to Medicinal Plants. Keats Publishing, 1977.
Shook, Edward Dr. Advanced Treatise on Herbology . Reprint Health Research.
Shosteck,Robert. Flowers and Plants. Quadrangle/The New York Times Book Co. 1974.
Siegfried, EV. Masters Thesis, Ethnobotany of the Northern Cree of Wabasca/Desmarais. U of Calgary, Alberta. 1994.
Silverman, Maida. A City Herbal. David R. Godine , 1990.
Silvertown, Jonathan. An Orchard Invisible. U of Chicago Press. 2009.
Simonot, Danielle. Bio-Manufacturing in Saskatchewan- Assessment of the Manufacturing Potential of Select Saskatchewan Plants, Sask. Nutraceutical Network, Saskatoon, 2000
Simpson, Brenan, M. Flowers At My Feet, Hancock House, Surrey, B.C. 1996.
Sionneau, P. An Introduction to the Use of Processed Chinese Medicinals. Blue Poppy Press, Second Printing 2003, Translated by Bob Flaws.
Smagghe, Guy Ed. Ecdysone. Structures and Functions. Springer Sci 2009.
Small, E & Catling, P. Canadian Medicinal Crops, NRC Research Press, Ottawa 1999.
Small, Ernest. Culinary Herbs, Second Ed. NRC Research Press, Ottawa, 2006.
_____ Medicinal Herbs, NRC Research Press, Ottawa, 2000.
_____ Top 100 Food Plants. NRC Press, Ottawa. 2009.
Smith, Andrew. Strangers in the Garden, the Secret Lives of Our Favorite Flowers.McClelland & Stewart 2004.
Smith, Annie Lorrain. Lichens, Cambridge at the University Press, 1921.
Smith, Harlan, Ethnobotany of the Gitksan Indians of B.C. Edited by B. Compton, B. Rigsby, and M.L. Tarpent, Mercury Series, Can Ethno Service, Paper 132, Can Mus of Civil. 1997.
Smith, Huron H. Manataka American Indian Council. www.manataka.org.
Snell, Alma Hogan. A Taste of Heritage. Crow Indian Recipes and Herbal Medicines. University of Nebraska Press 2006.
Soule, Deb. The Roots of Healing, A Woman's Book of Herbs. Citadel Press, 1995.
Spencer, Kate. The Magic of Green Buckwheat ,Richard Clay, England, 1987.
Spinella, Marcello. The Psychopharmacology of Herbal Medicine. MIT Press, 2001.
Steedman, E.V. The Ethnobotany of the Thompson Indians of British Columbia. 1930.
Stein, Sara. My Weeds, A Gardener's Botany. Harper and Row, 1988.
Stern, Gai. Australian Weeds. Harper and Row, Australia 1986
Stern Wm. Stern's Dictionary of Plant Names for Gardeners. Cassell Pub, London, 1972
Stewart, Hilary. CEDAR. Douglas & McIntyre. Vancouver/Toronto, 1984.
Storl, Wolf D. Healing Lyme Disease Naturally. NorthAtlantic Books, Berkeley, CA 2010.
Strehlow,W & Hertzka,G. Hildegard of Bingen's Medicine Bear & Co. Santa Fe 1988
Stuart, David. Dangerous Garden. Harvard University Press, Cambridge, Mass. 2004
Sturdivant L.&Blakley,T. Medicinal Herbs in the Garden, Field and Marketplace Bootstrap Guide, San Juan Naturals, Friday Harbor,WA, 1999.
Sumner, Judith. The Natural History of Medicinal Plants. Timber Press, Oregon, 2000.

Swanton, J.R. Haida Texts and Myths. Bureau Am Ethnol, Bull #29. Smithsonian Inst. Washington, D.C. 1905.
_____ Bureau of Am Ethno 26th Ann Report. Smithsonian Inst. Washington, 1908.
Szczeklik, Andrzej. Kore: On Sickness, the Sick and the Search for the Soul of Medicine. Counterpoint Berkeley 2012.
Tainter, D& Grenis A, Spices and Seasonings , VCH Pubishers, New York, 1993.
Talalaj,S.& Czechowicz,A S. Herbal Remedies, Hill of Content Press, Melbourne, 1989
Taylor, Wm &Farnsworth,N. The Vinca Alkaloids, Marcel Dekker, New York, 1973.
Teeguarden, Ron. The Ancient Wisdom of the Chinese Tonic Herbs. Warner Bros. 1998.
Telesco, Patricia. The Victorian Flower Oracle, Llewellyn Pub. St. Paul 1994
Temple, Robert. The Genius of China. Simon and Schuster. New York. 1986.
Thompson, Gerry, Astral Sex to Zen Teabags. Findhorn Press, 1994.
Thoreau, Henry David. Wild Fruits. W. W. Norton & Co. New York, 2000.
Throop, Priscilla. Hildegard von Bingen's Physica. Healing Arts Press, Vt. 1998.
Tick, Edward. The Practice of Dream Healing. Quest Books Wheaton, Illinois, 2001.
Tierra, Michael. The Way of Herbs- revised Pocket Rooks, New York, 1998.
Tigner, Daniel. Canadian Forest Tree Essences, self published,1998. ISBN 0968365809
Tilford, Gregory. Edible and Medicinal Plants of the West. Mountain Press, Missoula 1997.
Timbrook, Jan. Chumash Ethnobotany. St. Barbara Mus, Heyday Books, Berkeley Ca 2007.
Traill, E.C. Studies of Plant Life in Canada. A. S. Woodburn, Ottawa, 1885.
Traill, C. P. The Backwoods of Canada. McClelland and Stewart. Toronto. 1846.
Tobyn, G., Denham, A., Whitelegg, M. The Western Herbal Tradition. 2000 years of medicinal herbal knowledge. Churchill Livingstone Toronto 2011.
Toop, Edgar W & Williams, Sara. Perennials for the Prairies. U of A&Saskatchewan. 1991.
Treben, Maria. Health Through God's Pharmacy. Wilhelm Ennsthaler. 1982.
Tresidder, Jack. Symbols and Their Meaning. Friedman/Fairfax Pub. 2007.
Tucker A. & DeBaggio,T. The Big Book of Herbs. Interweave Press. Loveland CO. 2000.
_____ The Encylcopedia of Herbs. Timber Press, Portland. 2009.
Turkington, Carol. The Home Health Guide to Poisons and Antidotes, Facts on File 1994
Turner, Nancy J. Food Plants of Interior First Peoples. UBC Press, Vancouver, 1997.
_____ Food Plants of Coastal First Peoples. UBC Press, Vancouver, 1995.
_____ Plant Technology of First Peoples in B.C. UBC Press, Vancouver, 1998.
_____ et al. Thompson Ethnobotany. Memoir #3, Royal B.C. Museum, 1996.
_____ Plants of Haida Gwaii. Sononis Press, Winlaw, B.C. 2004.
_____ The Earth's Blanket. Douglas & McIntyre. Vancouver. 2005.
Turner, N & von Aderkas, P. Common Poisonous Plants and Mushrooms. Timber Press 2009
Turner, W.B. Fungal Metabolites, Academic Press, London and New York, 1971.
Twitchell, Paul. Herbs The Magic Healers. Eckankar, Box 3100 Menlo Park, CA, 1986.
Vermeulen, Nico. Encyclopedia of Herbs. Whitecap Books, Vancouver B.C. 1998.
Viereck, Eleanor, G. Alaska's Wilderness Medicines. Alaska Northwest Pub. 1987
Vitt, Marsh and Bovey, Mosses, Lichens, and Ferns, Lone Pine Press, 1988.
Vogel, A. Swiss Nature Doctor. A. Vogel, Switzerland. 1952
_____ Nature-Your Guide to Healthy Living. Verlag A. Vogel, Teufen, Switzerland 1986.
Vogel, Virgil. American Indian Medicine, U. of Oklahoma Press, Norman, 1970
Walker, Barbara. The Woman's Dictionary of Symbols&Sacred Objects. Csstle Books, 1988.
Walker, Marilyn. Wild Plants of Eastern Canada. Nimbus Pub. Halifax NS. 2008.
Ward, Bobby J. The Plant Hunter's Garden. Timber Press, Portland. 2004.
Ward-Harris, Joan.More Than Meets the Eye, The Life and Lore of Western Wildflowers Oxford University Press, Toronto, 1983

Watanabe & Shibuya. Pharmacological Research on Traditional Herbal Medicines. Harwood Academic Publishers, 1999.
Watt, John, and Breyer-Brandwijk, Maria The Medicinal and Poisonous Plants of Southern and Eastern Africa . E and S. Livingstone. Edinburgh and London. 1962.
Watts, Donald. Elsevier's Dictionary of Plant Lore. Elsevier. 2007.
Waugh, F.W. Iroquois Foods and Food Preparation #12 Anthropological Series, Ottawa. 1916. Reprinted by Iroqrafts, RR #2, Ohsweken, Ontario N0A 1M0, 1991.
Weaver, Wm. 100 Vegetables & Where They Came From. Workman Pub. New York, 2000.
_____ Sauer's Herbal Cures America's First Book of Botanic Healing 1762-1778, Routledge, New York, 2001.
Weed, Susan. Menopausal Years, The Wise Woman Way. Ash Tree Pub. Woodstock NY, 1992
Weigle, Marta. Spiders and Spinsters. U. of New Mexico Press, Albuquerque, 1982.
Weiner, M. The People's Herbal, A family guide. Putnam Publishing, New York, 1984.
Weiss, Rudolf. Herbal Medicine. Beaconsfield Publishers, 1988.
_____ Herbal Medicine 2nd Edition. Thieme, Stuttgart, New York, 2000.
Wells, Diana.100 Flowers and How They Got Their Names, Algonquin Books, Chapel Hill,97
Westcott, Frank. The Beaver Nature's Master Builder. Hounslow Press, Willowdale, ON '89.
Westrich, LoLo, California Herbal Remedies, Gulf Pub Co. Houston, TX, 1989.
Wetzel, Suzanne et al. Bioproducts from Canada's Forests. Springer Netherlands 2006.
WHO monographs on selected medicinal plants, vol 1, 1999; vol 2, 2002.
White, Ian. Australian Bush Flower Essences. Bantam Books, 1991
White, Florence. Flowers as Food . Jonathan Cape. 1934
Whitmont, Edward. Psyche and Substance. North Atlantic Books. 1980
Wilkinson, Kathleen. Trees and Shrubs of Alberta. Lone Pine Books, Edmonton 1990.
_____ Wildflowers of Alberta. U of A/Lone Pine Books, Edmonton 1999.
Williams, Jude. Nature's Gentle Cures. Sterling Publishing. New York. 1997.
Williamson, Darcy. 130 Medicinal Plant Monographs of the NW. self pub. E-book. 2011.
Williamson, E. Major Herbs of Ayurveda. Churchill Livingstone, Elsevier Science, 2002.
Winston, David. Herbal Therapeutics. HT Research Library Broadway NJ 8th Ed 2003.
_____ & Maimes, S. Adaptogens: Herbs for Strength, Stamina and Stress Relief. Healing Arts Press, Rochester, Vermont 2007
Wolf, Adolf Hungry, Teachings of Nature/Good Med Book,#14 Box 844 Invermere 1975.
Wolfson, Evelyn. From the Earth to Beyond the Sky. Houghton Mifflin Co. Boston, 1993.
Wood, Matthew. The Book of Herbal Wisdom. North Atlantic Books, Berkeley, 1997.
_____ Seven Herbs: Plants as Teachers, North Atlantic, Berkeley, 1986.
_____ Vitalism, the history of Herbalism, etc. N. Atlantic, Berkeley 1992.
_____ The Practice of Traditional Western Herbalism. N. Atlantic, Berkeley 2004.
_____ The Earthwise Herbal. Two vols. North Atlantic, Berkeley, 2008 and 2009.
Wood, Rebecca. The New Whole Foods Encyclopedia, Penguin Arkana, New York, 1999.
Worwood, Valerie. The Fragrant Heavens. New World Library. Novato CA, 1999.
Wren, R.C. Potter's New Cyclopaedia of Botanical Drugs and Prep. C.W. Daniel, 1988.
Wright, Clarrisa D. Food What We Eat and How We Eat . Ebury Press, London, 2000.
Wu, Jing-Nuan. An Illustrated Chinese Materia Medica. Oxford U Press. New York 2005.
Wulf-Tilford M. & G. All You Ever Wanted to Know About Herbs for Pets. BowTie Press, 1999
Yance Jr, D. Herbal Medicine, Healing and Cancer. Keats Publishing, Chicago, 1999.
Yang Shou-zhong. The Divine Farmer's Materia Medica. Blue Poppy Pr, Boulder, Co 1998.
Yang Xinrong. Encyclo Reference of Traditional Chinese Medicine. Springer Berlin 2003.
Yarnell, Eric et al. Clinical Botanical Medicine. Mary Ann Liebart Pub. NY 2002.
Yeager, S et al. New Foods for Healing. Prevention Health Books, Rodale Press, 1998.

Ying, Jianzhe, et al. Icones of Medicinal Fungi from China. Science Press, Beijing 1987
Young David et al. Cry of the Eagle, Encounters with a Cree Healer, U of Toronto Press, '89
Young, Jane & Hawley, Alex. Plants and Medicines of Sophie Thomas. 2nd Ed. 2004.
Yun, Henry. Herbal Holistic Approach to Arthritis. Dominion College. 1988.
Zevin, Igor V. A Russian Herbal. Healing Arts Press, Rochester, Vermont. 1997
Zheleznova, Irina. Northern Lights, Fairy Tales of the Peoples of the North, Progress Publishers, 1976.
Zinmeister & Mues. Bryophytes-Their Chemistry... Clarendon Press, Oxford, 1990.

FLOWER ESSENCE RESOURCES

Aditi Himalaya Flower Essences, 15,Jaybharat Society, 3rd Road, Khar (W), Bombay 400 052, India.

Alaskan Flower Essence Project, P.O. Box. 1369, Homer, Alaska USA 99603-1369. www.alaskanessences.com.

Australian Bush Flower Essences. Australia. www.ausflowers.com.au.

Bach- Healing Herbs English Flower Essences- in Canada by Self Heal Distributing, Box 95008, Whyte Postal Outlet, Edmonton, AB T6E 0E5, 1800-593-5956 or www.selfhealdistributing.com Also www.healingherbs.co.uk or www.fesflowers.com

Bailey Flower Essences, 8 Neslon Road, Ilkley, West Yorkshire England, LS298HN. www.flowervr.com

Bloesem Remedies. Netherlands. www.bloesem-remedies.com

BrynaHerb Essences. www.brynaherbessences.uk

Canadian Forest Essences, PO Box 29128,1996 W Broadway, Vancouver, BC V6J 1Z0

Canadian Forest Tree Essences. Ottawa. www.essences.ca. 613-725-9764.

Choming Flower Essences. www.mkprojects.com

Clear Path Essences. www.clearpathessences.com

Dancing Light Orchid Essences. Fairbanks, Alaska. www.orchidessences.com

Desert Alchemy, PO Box 44189, Tucson, Arizona, USA 85733. www.desert-alchemy.com.

Deva Flower Essences BP3 38880, Autrans, France. www.lab-deva.com

Eastern Flower Herbal Essences. julied@hfx.eastlink.ca.

Falling Leaf Essences. Box 78, Kallista, Victoria 3791, Australia. www.advancedalchemy.com.au.

Findhorn Flower Essences, Morayshire, Scotland IV36 0TY. www.findhornessences.com

Florais des Minas, Rua Albita, 194-Sala 408, Cruziero, CEP 30310-160,BH, MG, BRAZIL

FlorAlive®, Brent Davis. Contact info@floralive.com

FES Flower Essence Society, PO Box 1769, Nevada City, California, USA, 95959. www.fesflowers.com

Canadian Distributor- Self Heal Distributing, Box 95008, Whyte Postal Outlet, Edmonton, AB T6E 0E5 – www.selfhealdistributing.com

Green Hope Farm Flower Essences, PO Box 125, Meriden, New Hampshire USA 03770

Green Man Tree Essences. www.greenmantrees.demon.co.uk.

Habundia Flower Essences. c/o Peter Aziz. PO Box 90, Totnes, Devon, England TQ11 0YG.

Harebell Remedies. Scotland. ellie@harebellremedies.co.uk.

Hawaiian Gaia Flower Essences. www.gaiaessences.com

High Sierra Flower Essences. PO. Box 4275 Truclee, CA 96160.

holly.hsb@highoctavehealing.com

Horus Flower Essences- horus@floweressences.de.

Hummingbird Remedies, PO Box 50161, Eugene, Oregon, USA 97405

Icelandic Flower Essences. www.kristbjorb.is.

Jade Mountain Flower Essences, Box 125, Mountain Lakes, New Jersey USA 07046-0125

Korte Phi. www.PHIessences.com

Light Heart Essences. England. www.lightheartessences.co.uk.

Light Mountain Flower Essences, Michael A. Vertolli, 1-800-667-HERB.

Living Essences of Australia, Box 355, Scarborough, 6019, Perth, Australia. www.livingessences.com.au

Living Flower Essences, www.livingfloweressences.com . Rhonda Pallasdowney.

Master's Flower Essences, 14618 Tyler Foote Rd Nevada City, California, USA, 95959.
www.masteressences.com
Miriana fortem Flower Essences. www.mirianaflowers.com and info@miraflowers.com.
naturaSacredplay, PO Box 32, Buckhorn, New Mexico, 88025, (505-535-2255).
New Millenium Flower Essences of New Zealand. info@nmessences.com.
New Zealand New Perception Flower Essences, PO Box 60-127,Titirangi, Auckland 7, NZ
Pacific Essences, Box 8317, Victoria, B.C. V8W 3R9. www.pacificessences.com.
Pegasus Products, PO Box 228, Boulder, Colorado, USA 80306-0228. 1-800- 527-6104.
Perelandra, Box 3603, Warrenton, VA. 22186. www.perelandra-ltd.com
Petite Fleur Essence, 8524 Whispering Creek Trail, Fort Worth, Texas, USA 76134.
www.aromahealthtexas.com
Prairie Deva Flower Essences, Box 95008, Whyte Postal Outlet, Edmonton, AB T6E 0E5
1-(780) 433-7882. www.selfhealdistributing.com
Ravenworks- joni@ravenworksministries.org
Running Fox Farm PO Box 381,Worthington, Maryland USA 01098
Star Peruvian Flower Essences. Santa Barbara. www.starfloweressences.com
Stars of the Meadow, David Dalton, Lindisfarne Books, Mass. 2006.
Sun Essences. Norfolk, England. www.sunessence.co.uk
Sweetwater Sanctuary Essences. www.plantspirithealing.com
Tree Frog Farm Flower Essences. www.treefrogfarm.com
Whole Energy Essences, PO Box 285, Concord, Mass. 01742
Wild Rose Essences. www.wildrose.com
Woodland Essence, PO Box 206, Cold Brook, New York, USA 13324.

9055692R00151

Printed in Great Britain
by Amazon.co.uk, Ltd.,
Marston Gate.